Moyer's Fluid Balance:
A Clinical Manual

MOYER'S FLUID BALANCE:
A Clinical Manual

JOHN C. VANATTA, M.D.
Professor of Physiology
Southwestern Medical School of the University of Texas
Health Science Center, Dallas, Texas

MORRIS J. FOGELMAN, M.D.
Clinical Professor of Surgery
Southwestern Medical School of the University of Texas
Health Science Center, Dallas, Texas

Second Edition

YEAR BOOK MEDICAL PUBLISHERS, INC.
Chicago • London

Reprinted, April 1952

Second edition, 1976

Reprinted, May 1978

Library of Congress Catalog Card Number: 76-11368

International Standard Book Number: 0-8151-8962-1

To
Dr. Carl A. Moyer
physician, scientist, and an inspiring teacher

Preface to the Second Edition

The aim of this manual is to present a simple practical schema of diagnosis pertaining to fluid and electrolyte imbalances which can serve as a practical guide to the tentative selection of appropriate therapeutic measures. That was Doctor Moyer's statement of the aim of the original edition of this monograph, and it remains the aim of this edition.

Since the first edition in 1952, there have been many advances in the understanding of the physiology of fluid imbalance and therapy. It would be impossible to incorporate all of these in a monograph and still have a volume that could be easily carried in the pocket on the hospital wards. Therefore, the authors have chosen to omit discussions of diagnosis and treatment of special disturbances, such as surgical shock and burns. Also, diseases which are a combination of endocrine and electrolyte disturbances, such as primary diseases of the parathyroid glands or of the adrenal cortex, have been omitted.

Emphasis is placed on the clinical diagnosis of the patient using history, signs and symptoms, together with the support given by laboratory findings. The bibliographies at the end of each chapter are not comprehensive, but are intended to aid the reader in his supplemental reading.

One chapter is given to idealized case histories, together with an analysis of the diagnosis and initial management of each case. Such problem solving has been useful in introducing this subject to medical students who have had only a few lectures on the subject of water balance.

The authors hope that this book will give the reader a broad general background in the area of water balance, and then, as Doctor Moyer indicated in the first edition, stimulate students of medicine and surgery "to spend the laborious hours of careful study required to develop a real appreciation and understanding of the importance of the body's fluids to life."

The authors wish to thank Mrs. Elinor Reinmiller who not only checked the accuracy of the bibliographies of the chapters, but who is also a friend of long standing of both of the authors, and who gave us encouragement during the writing of the manuscript. We also thank Mrs. Trish Nickell who prepared all of the diagrams for this book.

JOHN C. VANATTA
MORRIS J. FOGELMAN

Preface to the First Edition

THE AIM of this manual is to present a simple practical schema of diagnosis pertaining to fluid and electrolyte imbalances which can serve as a practical guide to the tentative selection of appropriate therapeutic measures.

A brief critical evaluation is given of certain signs and symptoms associated with changes in the body's content of fluid and electrolytes.

The clinical manifestations of the common types of fluid and electrolyte derangements seen by the surgeon have been particularly stressed because laboratory data cannot adequately serve as the sole basis for fluid and electrolyte therapy. The major types of complications encountered in parenteral fluid therapy are also discussed.

The bibliographic references at the end of each chapter are not intended to be comprehensive. Many other important articles have provided ideas. Among these, the writings of A. M. Butler, W. M. Marriott, A. Blalock, H. Newburg, and F. P. Underhill are especially important.

I hope that this work will stimulate students of medicine, and more especially surgical residents, to spend the laborious hours of careful study required to develop a real appreciation and understanding of the importance of the body's fluids to life.

C. A. M.

Table of Contents

1 / The Chemistry of Body Fluids

THE WATER CONTENT of individuals is often stated to be 70% of the body weight. More accurately stated, it is approximately 70% of the body weight of a fat-free individual. The fatty tissue of an individual contains little water. This fatty tissue can vary from 10% to 40% of a person's body weight. This variation in fat content causes the water content of the body, when figured on the basis of total body weight, to vary from about 40% to 70%. The content averages about 60% for males 17 to 40 years of age, and 51% for females in the same age range. Therefore, 60% of the body weight will be used as a reasonable figure for total body water.

The composition of plasma, interstitial cell fluid, and intracellular fluid are presented in Figure 1–1.

The important points to make about the data presented in this figure are:

1. The values for plasma are the most reliable. Plasma is the body fluid most easily obtained in pure form for direct analysis.

2. The values for interstitial cell fluid are best obtained by calculation from the composition of plasma. The calculations assume that interstitial fluid is an ultrafiltrate of plasma. In ultrafiltration, the protein is removed, and the composition is changed in accordance with the principles of Donnan equilibrium.

3. The composition of cells is difficult to determine because the cells cannot be obtained in pure form. Problems of skeletal muscle analysis are explained in Chapter 2. Even packed red cells will have some fluid trapped between them when they are analyzed. Also, red cells are not typical body cells because their membranes are permeable to Cl^-.

4. Intracellular fluid is actually not a single pure fluid, but rather a weighted average value of the composition of fluid in nuclei, mitochondria, cytoplasm, and other cellular elements.

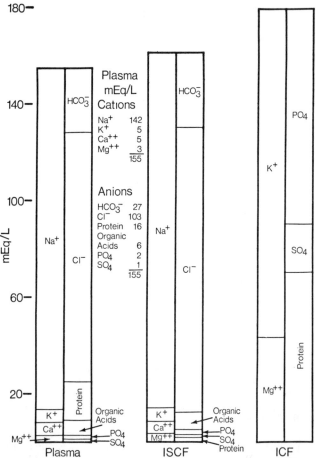

Fig 1–1.—The composition of plasma, interstitial cell fluid (*ISCF*), and intracellular fluid (*ICF*). The plasma values are obtained by analysis. The ISCF values were calculated from plasma, correcting for both the difference in water content and for Donnan equilibrium. Some published charts are corrected only for Donnan equilibrium. ICF values are best estimates from analyses. (Adapted from Gamble.)

UNITS OF MEASURE

The milliequivalent (mEq) is 1/1000 of an equivalent weight of an element or a compound. The milliosmole (mOsm) is 1/1000 of an osmole.

An equivalent weight of a substance is that weight of an element or compound which has the chemical-combining capacity equal to a gram-atomic weight of hydrogen ions. For example, a gram-atomic weight of chlorine (35.5 gm) will combine with a gram-atomic weight of hydrogen ions (1 gm). In turn, 39 grams of potassium will combine with 1 gram-atomic weight of chlorine, so that 39 grams is 1 equivalent weight of K. On the other hand, 1 gram-atomic weight of calcium (40 gm) will combine with 2 gram-atomic weights of chlorine. It follows then that an equivalent weight of calcium is 20 gm, which is one-half of its gram-atomic weight. (The equivalent weight is then the gram-atomic weight divided by the valence, which in the case of calcium is 2.)

An osmole of a substance is related not to its combining capacity but to its capacity to produce an osmotic pressure in solution. This depends upon the number of particles it produces per unit volume of solution. (Strictly speaking, it should be per unit volume of solvent, but for clinical work this difference is often disregarded. In some disease states, however, such as hyperlipoidemia, the distinction between the two ways of stating concentration is important.)

If 1 gram-molecular weight of a non-ionized substance is dissolved in 1 L of solution, the concentration is stated to be 1 osmolar. If it is dissolved in 1 kg of water, it is 1 osmolal. The osmotic pressure of either solution is approximately 22.4 atmospheres. Any solution which has an osmotic pressure equal to this is said to be 1 osmolar.

The osmotic pressure exerted by a substance in solution is dependent upon the number of particles per unit volume. It is not dependent upon the chemical-combining capacity of the substance. An osmole of the cationic, or anionic, portion of a completely ionized salt is its gram-atomic weight regardless of its valence. Thus, 23 gm of Na^+, or 40 gm of Ca^{++}, would constitute 1 osmole. In solution, the cation would of course be balanced by an anion, and so the total osmoles in a solution would be the sum of the cationic and anionic osmoles.

An osmole of a compound which is not ionized, such as dextrose, is its molecular weight. If a univalent compound such as NaCl is completely ionized, then there are 2 particles for each molecule, and 1 molecular weight constitutes 2 osmoles. If the monovalent compound is only partially ionized, then 1 osmole is some fraction of its molecular weight, that fraction being between 1/2 and 1, depending upon the degree of ionization.

Currently, most of the mathematics of converting analytic values from units of either milligrams per cent (mg %) or volumes per cent (vol %) is done by the clinical laboratory. A student of water balance should have available the mathematical formulas for converting from these units to mEq/L in order to read older literature. For this reason, Table 1–1 is presented giving the arithmetical steps for such conversions.

TABLE 1–1.—CONVERSION OF UNITS % TO mEq/L

SUBSTANCE			FUNCTIONAL VALENCE	ATOMIC WEIGHT	
Na^+	mg %	× 10	× 1	÷ 23	=
K^+	mg %	× 10	× 1	÷ 39	=
Ca^{++}	mg %	× 10	× 2	÷ 40	= mEq/L of plasma
SO_4^{--}	mg %	× 10	× 2	÷ 32	=
HPO_4^{--}	mg % as P	× 10	× 1.8	÷ 31	=
Cl^{-*}	mg %	× 10	× 1	÷ 35.5	=
CO_2 content	vol %	÷ 2.23	= mEq HCO_3/L of plasma		
Protein	gm %	× 2.43	= mEq/L of plasma		

*If the laboratory reports chloride as mg % NaCl, then the calculation is mg % × 10 × 1 ÷ 58.5 = mEq/L.

SERUM OR PLASMA CONCENTRATION

Whether serum or plasma is used for analysis is a technical problem which will not be discussed in detail. In general, analysis of serum and plasma do not give significantly different values for electrolytes except for potassium. In this case, plasma is preferred since potassium is likely to be released from the formed elements during the clotting process.

The subscript p is used throughout, to indicate plasma concentrations, even though the analysis might be done on serum.

BIBLIOGRAPHY

Gamble, J. L.: *Chemical Anatomy, Physiology and Pathology of Extracellular Fluid* (6th ed.; Cambridge: Harvard University Press, 1954).

2 / The System for Diagnosis

IT IS THE PURPOSE of this chapter to introduce the overall scheme for diagnosis of a case in which there is a disturbed water and electrolyte balance. Using this scheme, the clinician should make a diagnosis of the qualitative change in each of the following: (1) extracellular fluid volume; (2) extracellular fluid concentration; and (3) extracellular fluid composition. The diagnosis of extracellular fluid composition should again be divided into at least three parts. These are: (a) the acid-base state of the individual; (b) the K concentration of plasma; and (c) the Mg concentration of plasma.

Each of these five diagnoses is made independently of the other diagnoses. Treatment is then instituted on the basis of the combination of the five diagnoses.

This scheme was proposed by Dr. Carl Moyer. It has the advantage of simplicity. It is based on an understanding of basic physiology. Much new information has been published since he introduced these concepts. This new knowledge is incorporated into the scheme in this book.

THE FLUID COMPARTMENTS

The total body water can be subdivided into extracellular fluid (ECF) and intracellular fluid (ICF). For clinical diagnosis, a consideration of these compartments will usually suffice.

The ECF is subdivided principally into plasma and interstitial cell fluid (ISCF). In addition, there are minor compartments that are subdivisions of the ECF. Some of these are cerebrospinal fluid, intraocular fluid, fluid in the gastrointestinal tract, and fluid in the renal tubules. Changes in some of these minor compartments are occasionally of importance in the diagnosis and treatment of disturbed water-balance states. Such changes will be mentioned when they are applicable, but a detailed discussion of these compartments is omitted.

CHARACTERISTICS OF THE COMPARTMENTS

The ECF has the following important characteristics:

1. Volume
2. Concentration
3. Composition

The qualitative changes in these ECF characteristics have been well studied in most disease states. The signs and symptoms of the disturbances are well correlated with the changes in laboratory values. Volume, concentration, and composition can all be quantitated by laboratory procedures. However, the determination of volume is not easily done, and is a procedure reserved for clinical research laboratories.

The intracellular fluid, similarly, has the same three important characteristics: volume, concentration, and composition. Volume and composition of ICF can vary independently of the volume and composition of ECF.

Changes in ICF concentration are easily assessed. The measured concentration of the ECF will be the same as the concentration of the ICF. This is because water moves freely across cell membranes. It follows, then, that a difference in total ionic concentration of the ICF and ECF cannot exist for any appreciable period of time.

Changes in ICF volume are not readily measurable clinically. In order to measure this volume, one must first measure total body water. This is a difficult procedure. Simultaneously one must measure the ECF volume. The ICF volume is calculated as the difference between the two measured volumes. The ICF volume then has the combined errors of the two measurements.

Very little work has been done in measuring changes in ICF composition. The reasons for this become apparent if the problem of determining the composition of the ICF of skeletal muscle is considered. First, a biopsy of the muscle would have to be obtained. The total electrolyte content of the muscle would have to be determined. This total would include not only ICF but also the ECF in the biopsy material. Therefore, the volume and composition of the ECF in the biopsy would have to be determined, and subtracted from the total.

There is, then, a paucity of direct evidence regarding changes in ICF composition. This is unfortunate because such changes must be important in disease processes. If such changes could easily be determined, the clinician would be better able to treat patients with disturbed water and electrolyte balance.

ECF VOLUME

The normal ECF volume is estimated to be 20% of the body weight. For a 70-kg person, this is then 14 L of ECF. In disease states the value may be increased or decreased. An increase or decrease in volume gives specific signs and symptoms. These signs and symptoms, together with the history, enable the physician to diagnose the change in volume as a separate entity from a change in concentration, or composition, which may coexist. The treatment for the change in volume is also fairly specific.

ECF CONCENTRATION

The ECF concentration is defined as the ratio of ECF solutes to the ECF volume. It is best measured with an osmometer, which gives the ratio in milliosmoles per kilogram of water (mOsm/kg). Normal values for plasma are from 275 to 290 mOsm/kg. The concentration may be estimated from the total electrolyte concentration. This value in mEq/L is multiplied by 2 because of the ionization of the salts. This gives a value of about 300 to 310 mOsm/L. A physical chemist would explain the difference in the two values by a concept of the activity of the ions. For some reason, the ions do not exert their full activity in producing either an osmotic pressure or a depression of the freezing point during the measurement in the osmometer.

Because repetition is essential to learning, it must be emphasized here—and again later in the book—that a change in concentration can be due either to an increase in the amount of solute, or a decrease in the amount of water. Most often, a *change in water content* of the body *is responsible for a change in concentration of the body fluids.* A loss of water without a loss of solute results in an increase in concentration, and a gain of water without a gain of solute results in a decrease in concentration.

The diagnosis of concentration is made separately from the

diagnosis of ECF volume. Changes in concentration do cause changes in ICF volume, and are explained in Chapter 3.

ECF COMPOSITION

The changes in composition emphasized in this book are the acid-base states, K concentration, and Mg concentration. In addition, changes in organic acids, especially lactic acid, will also be discussed briefly.

The normal composition of ECF is portrayed by the bar graphs in Figure 1–1. A change in the composition of plasma without a change in total concentration is shown in Figure 2–1. In this example, the bicarbonate has increased from 27 to 36 mEq/L, with a concomitant decrease in chloride from 103 to 94

Fig 2–1.—A compositional change in plasma without a change in total concentration. The bicarbonate concentration has increased with a compensatory decrease in chloride concentration.

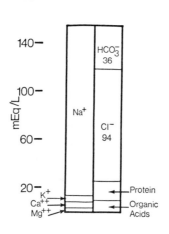

Plasma,   Compositional
Disturbance

mEq/L. The total ECF concentration is unchanged, i.e., 155 mEq/L.

The possible changes in composition are numerous. Technically, changes in the concentration of calcium, phosphate, sulfate, or proteins are changes in composition. However, this discussion will be limited to those changes just mentioned.

Although changes in ECF composition often coexist with changes in ECF volume and/or concentration, the changes are best considered separately in making the initial diagnosis.

EXAMPLE

An example of a diagnosis using this scheme would be:
ECF volume: slightly decreased
ECF concentration: markedly decreased
ECF composition
  Acid-base: compensated respiratory alkalosis
  Potassium: decreased
  Magnesium: normal

Having presented this scheme for making the diagnosis, we will emphasize in the rest of the book: (1) the methods for arriving at a correct diagnosis; and (2) the principles of treatment.

BIBLIOGRAPHY

Brozek, J. (ed.): Body composition, Ann. N.Y. Acad. Sci. 110:7-1018, 1963.

Moore, F. D., *et al.: The Body Cell Mass and Its Supporting Environment* (Philadelphia: W. B. Saunders, 1963).

3 / Milliosmolar Concentration Disturbances

THE UNDERSTANDING of the etiology of concentration disturbances embodies the understanding of water balance in its most literal sense, i.e., the gain and loss of water which contains no salt. In Moyer's scheme of diagnosis water is defined as a distinctly different entity from salt water. Salt water, unless otherwise qualified, refers to a solution containing salts at approximately isotonic concentration (155 mEq/L). Water refers to water containing virtually zero concentration of salts. By this definition most soft drinks, fruit juices, beer, and wine are considered—for water-balance purposes—as water. Likewise a dextrose solution in water, is water.

Occasionally, these classifications are not adequate to meet the situation. This is especially true when dealing with hypotonic salt solutions in the range of 30–125 mEq/L. Such solutions are encountered as losses chiefly in sweating, and will be discussed under this heading later in this chapter.

First, a discussion of normal water balance with the routes of gain and loss will be presented, and then the syndromes of simple water deficit and simple water excess will be discussed.

WATER BALANCE

The routes of, and a reasonable range of values for, normal water gain and loss are shown in Table 3–1. As indicated, over a 24-hour period water gain equals water loss. Within the 24-hour period, man continuously loses water from his body, but the principal routes of replacement occur intermittently.

Because of the intermittent replacement, it is difficult to precisely state when an individual has his "normal body content of water," with no excess and no deficit. There is evidence that most human beings achieve such a state when they eat a meal, and are allowed to take water ad lib.

Lower forms of animals, such as dogs, can be deprived of water and then allowed to drink. When they drink they will ingest just sufficient water to replace their deficit, and then

13

TABLE 3-1.—THE GAIN AND LOSS OF WATER

GAIN		LOSS	
Fluid intake	800–1,500	Urine	800–1,500
Water in food	475–725	Feces	125
Water of oxidation	250	Insensible loss	
		skin	250–375
		lungs	250–375
		Sweat	100
TOTAL GAIN	1,525–2,475	TOTAL LOSS	1,525–2,475

The routes, with reasonable normal values, are given for a 70-kg adult in an environment with moderate temperature and humidity, and no strenuous exercise. All values are in ml per 24 hours.

stop drinking. Man, if offered fluids in such a situation, will usually not replace his water loss completely. If he is given both food and liquids, he will completely replace his losses.

This is called a state of zero water load. Positive or negative water loads are measured from this point. The loads are best expressed as the percentage of the normal body weight of the individual. Thus, a person having a positive water load of 1% of his body weight would have an excess of water over his normal water content. In a 70-kg man, this would be 700 ml of water.

ROUTES OF GAIN

The intake of water in fluid form is obvious. It is important to realize that this is not the only route of gain. The volume taken in by this route can be difficult to evaluate when taking a history, even from an intelligent patient. People just do not pay that much attention to their habits of ingesting fluids.

In addition to the fluid intake, it must be remembered that most foods contain water. For example, raw meat is approximately 70% water. The water content of the meat will change, depending upon the method of cooking. If a patient takes no solid food, then the water normally ingested in the food must be replaced by an increased fluid intake.

A small quantity of water is formed from the oxidation of food. Even if a person has no food intake, he will burn stores of fat, protein, and/or carbohydrate. In the oxidation of these, water is formed.

ROUTES OF LOSS

Urine

The urinary loss of water in a normal person at moderate temperatures tends to change with the needs of the body to maintain normal concentration of the body fluids. It is, then, primarily dependent upon the total water gain. The regulation is through the osmoreceptors of Verney which control the release of the antidiuretic hormone (ADH) from the posterior pituitary. This hormone then regulates the volume and concentration of urine formed. The details of this regulation will not be covered in this book. If the reader is not familiar with these mechanisms, he may wish to read about them in a textbook on physiology or on renal function.

The regulation is so efficient in preventing a severe milliosmolar dilution in a normal person that it is virtually impossible to produce this disturbance by voluntarily increasing water intake. As increased volumes of fluids are drunk, the urine volume can increase to as much as 1.4 liters per hour in an adult.

On the other hand, this mechanism can be rather easily disturbed, so that it does not respond to a water excess. Surgery, pain, or a mild saltwater loss are some of the more common things which impair this regulatory mechanism.

If the rate of water gain is decreased, or is not sufficient to supply water needed for sweating in order to maintain body temperature, then the antidiuretic hormone and kidney will operate to reduce urine volume and, thereby, conserve water. In so doing, the kidney will not prevent a milliosmolar concentration from occurring, but will keep the urine loss of water from markedly contributing to the severity of a milliosmolar concentration.

The classic exception to this is diabetes insipidus, a disease state in which the kidney is the cause of a simple water deficit; if intake does not increase to match the water loss, a severe water deficit will ensue.

When the kidney does respond to a water deficit, the urine is not only small in volume, but also high in solute content. This produces a urine of high specific gravity. There are sufficient exceptions to this so that the finding of high specific gravity of the urine is of limited usefulness in the diagnosis of water deficit.

Insensible Loss (Lungs)

Expired air is at 100% relative humidity at body temperature. At a normal body temperature of 37 C, this water, which is in vapor form, is calculated to be the equivalent of 0.034 ml of liquid water per liter of air. If the inspired air were at 50% humidity at 25 C (a reasonable ambient temperature), the inspired air would contain water vapor equivalent to 0.011 ml of liquid water per liter of air. The difference in content of the expired air minus the inspired air represents a loss of pure water from the body. A reasonable value for this loss is 350 ml/day.

Viewed in this way, it can be appreciated that the rate of loss is increased by anything that increases the respiratory minute volume. An increase in body temperature also increases the amount that is contained in the expired air at 100% humidity. With fever and rapid breathing, the rate of loss can increase to 1,500 ml/day, or more.

This route of loss would be decreased to zero if the environmental temperature were body temperature, and the humidity were 100%. These environmental conditions are not likely to be encountered.

Insensible Loss (Skin and Sweating)

Insensible loss through the skin and sweating are technically different. From a clinical standpoint, it is convenient to consider them together. Often these will be added to the insensible loss from the lung and this total considered as a unit in discussing a patient's water-balance state.

Insensible loss through the skin occurs as water moves through the layers of the skin and escapes into the surrounding air in the form of water vapor. This loss is not related to the secretion of the sweat glands. Insensible loss occurs even in those rare individuals who have congenitally absent sweat glands. On the other hand, when sweating occurs, the surface of the skin becomes moist, and this true insensible loss from the skin then decreases to zero.

Sweat is always hypotonic. This will be discussed more thoroughly in Chapter 4. When the individual is acclimatized to heat, the $[Na^+]$ of sweat may be as low as 10 mEq/L. At this concentration, sweat is considered as a route of simple water loss. The sweat will contain potassium in concentrations of 5–10 mEq/L. The implications of this K^+ loss are discussed in Chapter 6.

The purpose of sweating is to supply water on the skin surface for evaporation. This evaporation causes a loss of heat from the body, and aids in the regulation of body temperature. The maximum rate of water loss by this route in an adult is 3.5 liters per hour.

Loss in Feces

The normal colon absorbs water from its contents so that the volume of water lost in feces is low. In addition, reabsorption of sodium and potassium is virtually complete. When a disease process disturbs the normal reabsorption, there is an increase in the volume of the stool, and it contains both salt and water. The loss is now a saltwater loss instead of a simple water loss.

PLASMA $[Na^+]$ COMPARED WITH OSMOLAL CONCENTRATION

In water deficit or excess, the diagnosis is aided by determining the ratio of total solutes to water in serum or plasma. If plasma is used, an anticoagulant must be chosen which will not disturb the ratio significantly. The most direct way of measuring this ratio is by osmometry. This method is based on the fact that solutes depress the freezing point of water in direct proportion to the number of particles in solution.

The reader will recall that certain physical properties of aqueous solutions depend upon the number of particles of solute present per unit weight of water. These are the colligative properties of solutions, and include both freezing-point depression and osmotic pressure. If one of these properties can be accurately determined, the other can be calculated. The osmometer, in effect, makes such a calculation. It is first calibrated with a solution of known osmolal concentration. The osmometer then electronically calculates the osmolal concentration of unknown from the freezing-point depression that it determines. The units are milliosmoles per kilogram of water.

Serum or plasma $[Na^+]$ is the next most useful index of the ratio of total solutes to water. It can be used as such an index because it constitutes over 90% of the total cations in plasma. The conditions under which this is useful, together with the common exceptions, are as follows:

1. The ratio of Na^+ to total cations is near the normal ratio of 142 mEq of Na^+ to 155 mEq of total cations.
2. The contribution of crystalloids to the total osmotic pressure is constant. Exceptions: hyperglycemia, azotemia.
3. The concentration of water in plasma is within normal limits, which is 92–93%. Exceptions: hyperproteinemia, hyperlipoidemia.

Since serum or plasma $[Na^+]$ is more commonly available than osmometry, it is useful to understand the basic physiological mechanisms by which the exceptions affect $[Na^+]_p$. If these are understood, then arithmetic corrections can be made so that $[Na^+]_p$ can still be used to evaluate the presence or absence of water excesses or deficits.

HYPERGLYCEMIA AND UREMIA

Both hyperglycemia and uremia reduce $[Na^+]_p$ by reason of their osmotic effects. Glucose or urea in effect replace the sodium salts so that the total osmotic pressure of plasma and ECF tends to remain normal.

For each rise of blood glucose of 180 mg % above the normal of 100 mg %, there is an increase in the osmotic pressure of plasma of 10 mOsm/L. This is calculated by using the molecular weight of glucose. If the total osmotic pressure remains in normal range, the concentration of the sodium salts must be reduced. Since the sodium salts are ionized, 1 mEq of sodium with its paired anion is equivalent to 2 milliosmoles of glucose. Therefore, for a rise of glucose to 280 mg % (180 mg % above normal), serum sodium would decrease 5 mEq/L if the total osmotic pressure remains normal. (If glucose rises suddenly, water may be drawn out of cells to dilute the sodium and there would be an increase in total osmotic pressure of both ECF and

ICF. If the rise is slow, both the renal and thirst mechanisms operate to maintain normal osmotic pressure.)

In summary:

$$\text{observed glucose} - 100 = \Delta\,G$$

where the units are mg % and $\Delta\,G$ is the increase in glucose concentration in plasma above normal.

$$\frac{\Delta\,G \times 10}{2 \times 180} = [\Delta\,Na^+]$$

where $[\Delta\,Na^+]$ is the expected decrease in $[Na^+]_p$ due to the increase in glucose.

For each rise in blood urea nitrogen (BUN) of 28 mg % above normal, there is an increase in osmotic pressure of 10 mOsm/L. Since a rise in nonprotein nitrogen (NPN) is chiefly due to a rise in urea nitrogen, the change in NPN could just as well be used for these calculations. The value is 28 because there are 28 mg of nitrogen in 1 milliosmole of urea. Again, as for glucose, since sodium is associated with an anion in plasma, such a rise would decrease $[Na^+]_p$ 5 mEq/L.

In summary:

$$\text{observed BUN} - 12 = \Delta\,U$$

or,

$$\text{observed NPN} - 25 = \Delta\,U$$

where the units are mg %, and $\Delta\,U$ is the increase in urea concentration in plasma.

$$\frac{\Delta\,U \times 10}{2 \times 28} = [\Delta\,Na^+]$$

where $[\Delta\,Na^+]$ is the expected decrease in $[Na^+]_p$ due to the increase in urea. This is then added to the observed $[Na^+]_p$ and the sum compared with normal values of $[Na^+]_p$ to evaluate the milliosmolar concentration of the plasma. If the sum is not within normal limits, then a disturbance in milliosmolar concentration probably exists.

Hyperproteinemia and Hyperlipoidemia

Hyperproteinemia and hyperlipoidemia lower plasma sodium by a different mechanism than elevated glucose and urea concentrations. To understand this mechanism, one must also understand that the important measurement here is the ratio of solutes to water, rather than the ratio of solutes to total plasma. In most cases, the relationships between these two values are so constant that it makes no difference which of the two concentrations is considered. Since the laboratory measures and reports sodium in mEq/L of plasma, it is simply convenient to use the plasma values.

Normal plasma is only 92% water. To state that there are *142 mEq of sodium per liter of plasma* really means that there are *142 mEq of sodium in 920 ml of water*. The other 80 ml is the volume occupied by the proteins, lipids, and crystalloids. Most of this remainder is protein, and sodium is not contained within the protein molecule. To determine the concentration of sodium *per liter of plasma water,* calculate:

$$142 \text{ mEq/L plasma} \div \frac{0.920 \text{ L water}}{1.0 \text{ L plasma}} = 154 \text{ mEq/L water}$$

In most disease states the concentration of water in plasma does not change, so that the 142 m/Eq/L plasma is satisfactory for diagnosis in most patients. However, when either hyperlipoidemia or hyperproteinemia occur, the water content of plasma may be reduced sufficiently to cause the wrong conclusions from a determination of sodium concentration of plasma.

For example, take an actual extreme case from the literature. This is a diabetic who had lipoidemia. The lipids in his plasma occupied so much space that the water content fell to 73%. The sodium concentration of the water was determined to be 141 mEq/L of water, a moderately reduced value. However, since there was only 730 ml of water per liter of plasma, the sodium concentration of plasma was only 103 mEq/L. If the cause of the low $[Na^+]_p$ were not recognized, errors in treatment of his water-balance state would result.

Similarly, elevated protein may displace plasma water and lower plasma sodium. However, it does not produce as severe a disturbance as the hyperlipoidemia just noted, because such a severe hyperproteinemia does not occur.

When a low sodium concentration occurs in a patient with hyperlipoidemia or hyperproteinemia, it is best to determine the concentration of solutes in mOsm/kg of water using an osmometer. If this determination is not available, the physician can estimate the effect of the lipids and protein on the $[NA^+]_p$ by the calculations that follow.

First, estimate the water content of plasma:

$$\text{water content} = 99.1 - 0.73\ P - 1.03\ L$$

where P is protein in gm/100 ml, and where L is lipids in gm/100 ml. The 0.73 comes from the volume occupied by 1 gram of protein; the 1.03 is the volume occupied by 1 gm of lipid. Water content is in units of the per cent water in plasma.

When the water content is calculated, each percentage unit that is below 92 will then lower plasma sodium by 1.5 mEq/L. This figure is a satisfactory approximation for clinical work.

THE NORMAL YANNET-DARROW DIAGRAM

The relationships between the changes in volumes and concentrations of ECF and ICF are easily diagrammed by using two rectangles representing ECF and ICF, as shown in Figure 3–1. This diagram was first introduced by Yannet and Darrow and carries their names.

In the diagram, the volume of the intracellular and extracellular compartments is proportional to the horizontal dimension of the respective rectangles. The milliosmolar concentration is proportional to the height of each rectangle. The areas, then, represent the total osmotically active solutes in the respective compartments.

The vertical line between the two rectangles represents the plasma membranes which separate the ECF from the ICF. Since all cells (except for a few such as the epithelial cells of the distal nephron) are freely permeable to water, any disequilibrium of concentration between ICF and ECF can exist only briefly because there will be a net water movement in response to the concentration difference and this will equalize the concentrations.

Normal Volume And Concentration

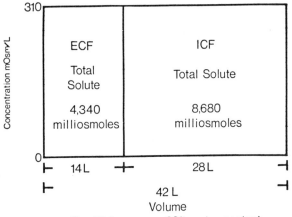

For 70-kg person, 60% water content

Fig. 3–1.—This diagram shows the relationships between the milliosmolar concentrations and volumes of the extracellular fluid (*ECF*) compartment and the intracellular fluid (*ICF*) compartment. The area of each compartment is the product of concentration times volume and represents the total solute in the compartment. Diagrams of this type were first used by Yannet and Darrow and bear their names.

MILLIOSMOLAR DILUTION

A simple water excess is produced in an individual by a rate of gain of water in excess of the rate of loss. The extra water dilutes the solutes, and a milliosmolar dilution results.

If a normal individual is subjected to surgery, or to a mild saltwater deficit, then a water excess may be easily produced by excess intake. The antidiuretic hormone and kidney mechanism no longer quickly respond to the water gain. When there is a water excess and saltwater loss combined, this state is more properly called a relative water excess. Treatment of the water excess in either case is similar, and differences will become apparent when the reader is introduced to the treatment of combined states in Chapter 7.

Synonyms: water excess, water intoxication, ICF volume excess, dilution syndrome, reduced milliosmolar concentration, inappropriate production of ADH.

Basic Dynamics

When water is ingested, or when 5% glucose in water is given intravenously, the water first enters the ECF compartment and dilutes the concentration of the electrolytes. (In the case of the glucose, the sugar is eventually removed from the ECF.) The osmotic gradient produced between ECF and ICF promptly causes the water to enter into the cells. The milliosmolar concentrations of ICF and ECF are equally reduced. This state is diagrammed in Figure 3–2.

It is not the reduction in concentration that gives rise to the more important signs and symptoms. Instead, it is the increase in volume of the intracellular fluid and, particularly, the increase in volume of the cells of the brain.

When water moves into the cells, the cells swell. In tissue such as skeletal muscle this is of little consequence. When the cells of the brain swell, this produces an increase in intracranial pressure because the brain is in an enclosed space with a fixed volume.

As the severity of the water excess and hence the swelling of the cells increases, a progression of symptoms occurs: headache, muscle twitching, convulsions with intervening stupor, and death. In addition, the increase in intracranial pressure may cause papilledema. The production of this depends not only on the intensity, but also the duration, of the water excess. It takes 24–48 hours for papilledema to develop in response to the increase in intracranial pressure.

The mechanism of production of the papilledema is compression of the retinal vein with resultant increase in venous pressure in the retina. This then raises capillary pressure in the retina until the hydrostatic pressure exceeds the oncotic pressure of plasma. Papilledema results.

In addition, the increase in intracranial pressure usually produces an elevation of systemic blood pressure. Teleologically, this serves to maintain the perfusion pressure of the brain. For the details of the physiological mechanism by which this is produced, the reader is referred to a standard basic physiology text.

Milliosmolar Dilution

Net gain of 4.2L H_2O

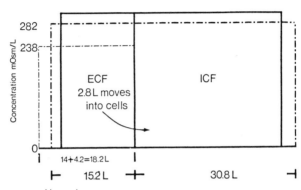

— Normal
--- All 4.2L H_2O gain in ECF
-·· Final state after osmotic equilibrium

Fig 3–2.—These composite diagrams show the relationships of the volumes and concentrations of the ECF and ICF when a normal individual gains 4.2 liters of water. Since there is no gain of solute, the area of each compartment must not change. The water first enters the ECF compartment and dilutes the osmotic concentration. This produces a disequilibrium and water quickly moves into the ICF. At equilibrium the concentrations of both compartments are equal, but lower than the normal value of 310 mOsm/L. The volumes of both compartments are increased proportionately.

CLINICAL PICTURE OF DECREASE IN OSMOLAR CONCENTRATION OF ECF

History
    A. Headache
    B. Nausea and vomiting
    C. Blurred vision
Physical Examination
    A. Neuromuscular apparatus (in order of appearance
       with increasing severity of the disturbance)
       1. Muscle twitching
       2. Hyperactive tendon reflexes

     3. Convulsions with stupor between convulsions
     4. Loss of reflexes

B. Signs of increased intracranial pressure
     1. Elevated cerebrospinal fluid pressure
     2. Projectile vomiting
     3. Hypertension
     4. Bradycardia
     5. Papilledema (after 24–48 hours)
     In severe water excess, the hypertension may be replaced by hypotension, and then tachycardia is more likely.

C. Signs of extrarenal water loss
     1. Moist mucous membranes with lacrimation
     2. Salivation
     3. Diarrhea

D. Fingerprint edema
     This is a reliable sign of water excess. The sign is demonstrated by the examiner firmly pressing his finger over the sternum (or other bony surface) for a period of 15–30 seconds. On removal of the finger, a positive sign consists of the examiner being able to see a recognizable fingerprint, similar to that which is made on paper with fingerprinting ink. The difference between this and soft-pitting edema is quite marked.

Laboratory findings

A. Blood and plasma
     1. Milliosmolal concentration as measured by an osmometer is decreased.
     2. $[Na^+]_p$ is decreased. If hyperglycemia, azotemia, hyperlipoidemia, or hyperproteinemia is present, the $[Na^+]_p$ must be corrected for the effects of these abnormalities before interpreting it with respect to milliosmolar concentration.

B. Urine
     1. Volume
     Initially as the osmolar concentration decreases, urine volume tends to increase, but eventually oliguria and anuria obtain. The kidney is unable to maintain normal osmolar concentration in the presence of water overload in the critically ill patient.
     2. Urine specific gravity is most often low.
     3. Urine chloride is most often low.

Other laboratory findings are of little value in diagnosis.

TREATMENT

Water should be withheld. If the milliosmolar dilution is mild, this may be sufficient therapy, since insensible loss will raise the concentration.

Hypertonic salt solutions may be given. They are indicated if the patient is convulsing, or has convulsed. When given, they should be administered in small quantities, and the effect carefully monitored. Five or six milliliters of 5% NaCl solution per kilogram body weight will raise the ECF $[Na^+]$ about 10 mEq/L.

If the patient is alkalotic, give 3% or 5% sodium chloride solution.

If the patient is in normal acid-base balance, give a mixture of hypertonic sodium chloride and sodium lactate.

In the presence of acidosis, 1/2 or 1 M sodium lactate may be utilized. Hypertonic $NaHCO_3$ has been utilized, but its use is not recommended because it can convert an acidosis into an acute alkalosis.

INCREASED MILLIOSMOLAR CONCENTRATION

Synonyms: water deficit, free-water deficit (when due to water loss); hyperosmolal hyperglycemia (when due to diabetes mellitus); solute-loading hyperosmolality, solute-loading hypertonicity, hyperalimentation (when due to overloading with solutes); ICF volume deficit.

An increase in milliosmolar concentration can be due to a net water loss or to a marked increase in solute content of the body. The evaluation of a net water loss is primarily the responsibility of the attending physician. He must consider these questions in making the evaluation:
1. How long has the patient been ill?
2. What is the environmental temperature?
3. Does the patient have fever which would increase the loss?

Obvious causes of decreased water intake that are frequently encountered are unconsciousness and dysphagia. Loss of water, in addition to that from insensible loss, may be from the kidney in diabetes insipidus. Alcoholics also develop water deficits by diuresis because ethanol inhibits the secretion of antidiuretic hormone.

A marked increase in solutes can occur in diabetes mellitus, and cause an increase in milliosmolar concentration. Associated with this is usually a glycosuria which causes a loss of both water and salt. The loss of water may exceed the loss of salt, and thus add to the increase in milliosmolar concentration.

Marked increases in solute concentration can occur because of increased ingestion of solutes. The drinking of sea water, which is hypertonic, would be an example of this. Iatrogenic overloading with solutes has occurred from administering nasogastric feedings which not only have salts in them, but also proteins and carbohydrates. If these are not matched with adequate water intake, hyperosmolality of body fluids will result. Similarly, this condition has occurred in infants when the formula is made incorrectly.

Patients with bleeding peptic ulcers may receive frequent feedings of milk and cream. They must also be given adequate quantities of water. It is possible that not only the milk and cream contribute solutes, but also that the partially digested blood is reabsorbed. Whole blood is isotonic, but when partially digested it appears that the polypeptides and other digested products contribute to an increase in the osmolality.

BASIC DYNAMICS

The basic dynamics of fluid movements in a simple water deficit are shown in Figure 3–3. Water is initially lost from the ECF compartment. This concentrates the solutes in the ECF, creating an osmotic gradient which causes water to shift from the ICF to the ECF. When osmotic equilibrium is established, the osmotic concentration of both compartments is increased and the volume of each is proportionately decreased.

If the milliosmolal concentration were produced by an increase in total solutes, then a similar movement of water out of the ICF would occur, but the ECF volume would be expanded. A solute excess can both increase the milliosmolar concentration and decrease the ICF volume quickly. In

Milliosmolar   Concentration

Net loss of 4.2 L H₂O

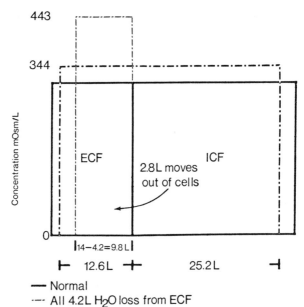

— Normal
·—· All 4.2L H₂O loss from ECF
···· Final state after osmotic equilibrium

Fig 3–3.—These composite diagrams show the relationships of the volumes and concentrations of the ECF and ICF when a normal individual has a net loss of 4.2 liters of water. Since there is no loss of solute, the area of each compartment must not change. Initially the loss is from the ECF and the osmotic concentration increases, but water moves from the ICF into the ECF to establish equilibrium. At equilibrium the concentrations of both compartments are equal, but higher than the normal value of 310 mOsm/L. The volumes of both compartments are reduced proportionately.

autopsy cases, cerebral hemorrhage is a frequent finding. Experiments on animals indicate the probable mechanism is a decrease in volume of the brain cells as ICF is drawn out, and a resultant decrease in intracranial pressure. The intracranial vessels then dilate and rupture. In addition, bridging veins are torn.

Cerebral thrombosis has been found in deaths due to solute excess. The pathological physiology which causes this is obscure.

CLINICAL PICTURE OF INCREASE IN OSMOLAR CONCENTRATION OF ECF

History
- A. Deprivation of water and food
- B. Possible increase in environmental temperature or body temperature
- C. Severe thirst. (This may be a symptom in other conditions.)
  or
- D. Diabetes mellitus with hyperglycemia
  or
- E. Hyperalimentation

Physical Examination
- A. Fever (if room temperature is above 65 F)
- B. CNS signs
  1. Moderate elevation in concentration
     a. Restlessness and weakness
  2. Severe elevation in concentration
     a. Lethargic and listless when undisturbed. (If stimulated, the patient often becomes irritable and hyperreactive.)
     b. Disorientation, delusions, and hallucinations
- C. Tissue signs
  1. Tongue dry and swollen
  2. Dry mouth
  3. Cutaneous erythema
  4. Viscera that stick to the gloved hand of the surgeon
- D. Renal signs
  Oliguria or anuria

E. Cardiovascular signs
   1. Increased blood pressure and pulse pressure early
   2. Tachycardia
   3. Hypotension in severe cases

Laboratory Findings
   A. Plasma
      1. Osmolality is increased as measured by an osmometer.
      2. $[Na^+]_p$ is increased.
      3. Sum of $[Cl^-]_p$ plus $[HCO_3^-]_p$ is increased.
      4. Protein concentration is usually increased, but normal concentration does not rule out this condition.
   B. Blood
      1. Red cell count may be elevated.
      2. $[Hb]$ may be increased.
   C. Urine
      1. Specific gravity is elevated, unless diabetes insipidus is the cause of the water loss.
      2. Red cells, casts, and albumin are often present.

TREATMENT

The treatment of hyperosmolality due to water deficit is clearly to administer water. In mild cases, water may be given by mouth, but in severe cases 5% glucose in water should be given intravenously since patients will tend to vomit water taken by mouth. In severe hyperosmolality, the rate of administration must not be too fast as it is possible to cause convulsions in the patient. Apparently there are compensations for the decrease in volume that takes place in the intracranial cavity, and reexpansion of the brain must not occur too rapidly. The replacement of the water deficit should be done gradually over about 48 hours.

Estimates of the volume of water needed and the rates of administration are not intended to replace careful evaluation of the individual patient during therapy. In a moderate disturbance in a 70-kg patient, 3 liters of 5% glucose in water can usually be given intravenously in 3–6 hours. In a disturbance severe enough to produce a semicomatose state, 4–6 liters of 5% glucose in water can be given to a 70-kg individual over a 24-hour period.

A method for estimating the water needs of a patient from the $[Na^+]_p$ is presented in Chapter 7.

If the hyperosmolality is a complication of diabetes mellitus, with a depressed $[Na^+]_p$, then different principles apply. The treatment of such a disturbance is difficult and the mortality is high. It must be remembered that insulin therapy will lower the glucose level, and thus reduce the osmotic pressure of the ECF. Water will then move into the ICF. Certainly, 5% glucose in water should not be given initially. Insulin is probably the best treatment of the osmotic disturbance in this special situation, and isotonic salt solution should be given if there is evidence of an ECF volume deficit.

Treatment of hyperosmolality due to solute excess varies with the severity of the excess. In mild cases, the same principles should be applied as for hyperosmolality due to a water deficit. Therapy of severe cases is difficult. If any degree of hypotension is present, then a solution which expands the vascular volume is desirable, such as plasma or a plasma substitute. At the same time, water should be given orally or rectally, if possible, or 5% glucose in water should be given intravenously to correct the osmolal disturbance. Again the rate of correction should be slow. It should be given over at least a 48-hour period, and possibly over 72 hours.

BIBLIOGRAPHY

Abele, J. E.: The physical background to freezing point osmometry and its medical-biological applications, Am. J. Med. Electronics 2:32, 1963.

Albrink, M. J., *et al.:* The displacement of serum water by the lipids of hyperlipemic serum. A new method for the rapid determination of serum water, J. Clin. Invest. 34:1483, 1955.

Bartter, F. C.: The Syndrome of Inappropriate Secretion of Antidiuretic Hormone (SIADH), in Dowling, H. F. (ed.): *Disease-A-Month* (Chicago: Year Book Medical Publishers, Inc., November, 1973).

Danowski, T. S., Fergus, E. B., and Mateer, F. M.: The low salt syndromes, Ann. Intern. Med. 43:643, 1955.

Finberg, L.: Hypernatremic Dehydration, in Schulman, I. (ed.): *Advances in Pediatrics,* vol. 16 (Chicago: Year Book Medical Publishers, Inc., 1969).

Jacobson, M. H., *et al.:* Urine osmolality, a definitive test of renal function, Arch. Intern. Med. 110:83, 1962.

Leaf, A.: The clinical and physiological significance of the serum sodium concentration, N. Engl. J. Med. 267:24, 1962.

Marriott, H. L.: Water and salt depletion, Br. Med. J. 1:245, 285 and 328, 1947.

Rowntree, L. G.: Water intoxication, Arch. Intern. Med. 32:157, 1923.

Sament, S., and Schwartz, M. B.: Severe diabetic stupor without ketosis, S. Afr. Med. J. 31:893, 1957.

Schoolman, H. M., Dubin, A., and Hoffman, W. S.: Clinical syndromes associated with hypernatremia, Arch. Intern. Med. 95:15, 1955.

Wolf, A. V.: *Thirst: Physiology of the Urge to Drink and Problems of Water Lack* (Springfield, Ill.: Charles C Thomas, 1958).

Wright, H. K., and Gann, D. S.: Hyperglycemic hyponatremia in nondiabetic patients, Arch. Intern. Med. 112:344, 1963.

Zimmermann, B., and Wangensteen, O. H.: Observations on water intoxication in surgical patients, Surgery 31:654, 1952.

4 / Extracellular Fluid Volume Disturbances

THE EXTRACELLULAR FLUID VOLUME is estimated to be 20% of the body weight. Actually, this percentage varies from individual to individual, depending upon the fat content of the body. Although it is accurate in concept to think of the ECF volume, the exact measurement of this volume is virtually impossible. The volume consists of all the fluid outside the cells. This would include not only interstitial cell fluid, but also cerebrospinal fluid, intraocular fluid, lymph, secretions present in the gastrointestinal tract, and fluid in the renal tubules.

In clinical research the investigator estimates ECF volume by measuring the distribution of a substance. An easily identifiable substance that distributes itself only in the ECF is injected. Radioactive sulfate is such a substance. A measured amount is injected, and its concentration in the plasma is measured after a suitable mixing time. From the dilution of the injected material a volume is calculated which is called a "space." Commonly measured spaces are those for sodium, inulin, sulfate, and chloride. Of these, the inulin and sulfate spaces are the smallest (about 16% of body weight) and they are probably the best indices of the true ECF volume.

In this chapter the physiology and diagnosis of alterations in ECF volume will be discussed.

EXTRACELLULAR FLUID DEFICIT

Synonyms: extracellular fluid volume deficit, saltwater loss, sodium deficiency. (Dehydration is not a good synonym because it is not specific. It does not distinguish between a saltwater loss and a simple water loss.)

One distinction must be made between the terms *extracellular fluid volume deficit* and *saltwater loss*. A saltwater deficit will always cause a decrease in ECF volume, and this very quickly becomes discernible clinically. A decrease in ECF volume, with all the signs and symptoms indicated, can occur in a very severe simple-water deficit. A simple-water deficit (see

Chapter 3) reduces the ECF and ICF volumes proportionately. The symptoms due to the concentration of body fluids usually cause the patient to seek help before the decrease in ECF volume shows prominent manifestations.

ROUTES OF LOSS

All secretions into the gastrointestinal tract are approximately isotonic. When these are lost from the body, there is a loss of salt in proportion to water and, therefore, a reduction in the ECF volume. Since salt is lost in proportion to water, there is *no change in the concentration of the extracellular fluid.*

Sodium may be lost in sweat. The concentration of sodium in sweat is quite variable, ranging from 9 to 80 mEq/L. If an individual loses 2 liters of sweat containing 75 mEq/L of Na^+, this is equivalent to losing 1 liter of isotonic salt solution and 1 liter of simple water. The salt loss will then decrease that individual's ECF volume.

One of the chief factors determining the $[Na^+]$ in sweat is whether or not the individual is acclimatized to heat. An individual who is not acclimatized to heat will have a higher $[Na]$ in his sweat than the individual who is acclimatized. As a result of this, an ECF volume deficit is more likely to occur in an individual who is suddenly changed from a cold to a warm environment. The incidence of this disturbance due to sweating is highest during the first 2 or 3 days of hot weather. Individuals who work in a very warm environment (such as around an open-hearth furnace) during mild or cold weather often have symptoms due to a saltwater deficit.

If an individual is subjected to warm temperatures continuously so that his environmental temperature does not drop below 70 F even at night, he will quickly acclimatize, and his salt loss in sweat is then virtually zero.

Salt water may be taken from the functional extracellular fluid space without being lost from the body. This is called a distributional shift in the ECF volume. Examples of this are:
1. Rapidly developing ascites. The peritoneal fluid is isotonic, and is similar in composition to interstitial cell fluid. If the ascites develops slowly, the individual usually will retain sodium from his diet. The rate of retention of sodium can then keep pace with the rate of movement of sodium into

the peritoneal cavity. If, on the other hand, the rate of formation of the ascites is quite rapid, then a severe ECF deficit is likely to occur. As the salt moves into the peritoneal cavity with the fluid, it must come from other parts of the body, and thereby deplete the ECF volume.

2. Small bowel obstruction. In small bowel obstruction, there is an accumulation of isotonic fluid in the lumen of the gut.
3. Peritonitis.
4. Burns.
5. Crushing injuries.

In examples 3, 4, and 5, edema occurs. This edematous fluid contains sodium and, technically, an excess ECF in the part involved. The salt and water in this fluid are drawn there at the expense of the ECF volume of normal tissue elsewhere in the body. The ECF volume deficit then occurs in these other normal tissues.

As an example of the magnitude of volume of ECF involved, consider a theoretical patient with severe sunburn over 0.9 fractional part of his body surface area. A reasonable surface area for an average adult is 2.0 square meters. If the skin were to increase in thickness by 0.3 cm by reason of the edema fluid, the volume of fluid would be calculated as follows:

total surface area × fraction burned × thickness =   volume
20,000 cm² ×   0.9   ×   0.3 cm   = 5,400 cm³

This volume is over 35% of an average person's ECF volume. The 0.3 cm thickening may be more or less, depending upon the severity of the burn.

Two occult routes of sodium loss are the following:

1. Drinking water, followed by vomiting. When water enters the stomach, sodium chloride and other electrolytes enter this water. The water must become nearly the same concentration as ECF fluid with respect to its salt content before any volume is absorbed. If the patient retains the water for a short period of time, and then vomits, there is a net loss of salt. The kidney usually will gradually correct the decrease in sodium concentration of the body fluids that is due to sodium salts having moved from the ECF into the stomach contents.
2. Subcutaneous administration of fluids. When dextrose in

water is given subcutaneously, it is not immediately absorbed into the circulation. Salts must first move into this fluid, and this movement continues until the concentration of sodium and the other electrolytes in the injected fluid is nearly that of normal ECF. This movement of salt out of the plasma causes a net dilution of the plasma and the ECF in other parts of the body. Such dilution persists only momentarily because water then moves into the cells by reason of the osmotic gradient that is established. As a result, there is a decrease in the ECF volume elsewhere in the body. This decrease will persist until the injected fluid is finally absorbed. The process of movement of salts and absorption takes several hours. In an individual who already had a decrease in ECF volume, the further decrease caused by the subcutaneous injection of dextrose in water could conceivably cause his demise.

BASIC PHYSIOLOGIC DISTURBANCES

Cardiovascular

When the ECF volume is decreased, the plasma volume is reduced. The osmotic pressure exerted by the plasma proteins serves to retain fluid in the vasculature. Therefore, a 20% decrease in ECF volume will usually result in less than a 20% decrease in plasma volume.

The decrease in plasma volume decreases total blood volume and this, in turn, decreases cardiac output. The disturbances in blood pressure and the poor filling of veins below a venous tourniquet are directly related to these events.

Decrease in Skin Turgor

In ECF volume deficit there is a decrease in skin turgor. When the skin of the forearm (or leg, abdomen, thorax, or back) of a normal individual is picked up and then released, it returns to the normal position in less than a second. In a patient with ECF volume deficit, there is a lack of quick return of the skin to its previous degree of flatness. The more severe the deficit, the slower the return.

The authors are not aware of any studies about the mechanism producing this stickiness of the skin. It seems reasonable that the intercellular space of the subcutaneous tissue is reduced and that, therefore, the cells do not move as easily over each other.

A decrease in skin turgor may occur without a saltwater deficit in the very elderly or in individuals who have had an extreme and rapid weight loss due to either dieting or severe illness.

Laboratory Findings

The laboratory findings of ECF volume deficit are conspicuous by their absence.

There are no common laboratory findings which are pathognomonic of ECF volume deficit. If measurements of sulfate space, inulin space, or any of the other spaces which estimate ECF volume were available, they would be reduced.

Measurements of plasma sodium and red cell concentrations are of minimal value but should be considered.

Plasma Na^+.—If salt is lost in proportion to water, then the $[Na]_p$ will remain normal. If the sodium concentration is changed, and there is a saltwater loss, then the concentration change indicates a concomitant change in simple water content. A high $[Na]_p$ indicates a simple water deficit, and a low $[Na]_p$ indicates a simple water excess. (Exceptions to these interpretations are noted in Chapter 3.)

Measurements of red cell concentrations.—The values of hematocrit, $[Hb]$, and red cell count all tend to be high in volume deficits. This is due to the decrease in plasma volume. It is, however, not advisable to rely upon these changes for either diagnosis or for assessing the magnitude of the deficit. If the volume of ECF decreases slowly, the body will decrease the red cell mass so that the ratio of red cell volume to plasma volume tends to remain normal. Even in an acute ECF volume depletion, where any of these three values would be expected to increase, they may be of little significance unless previous values are also available for the given patient. For example, it would be difficult to tell whether a single determination of $[Hb]$ of 15 gm/100 ml is normal for that patient or whether it represents a change from a low normal of 12 gm/100 ml to 15 gm/100 ml. Such a change is theoretically caused by a 25–30% decrease in plasma volume.

CLINICAL PICTURE OF ECF VOLUME DEFICIT WITHOUT SIGNIFICANT CHANGE IN OSMOLAR CONCENTRATION

History
  A. Rapid loss of body fluids without sodium intake, or burns, crushing injury, or peritonitis
  B. Weakness
  C. Dizziness on sitting or standing
  D. Syncope
Physical Examination
  A. Signs of depressed CNS activity
     1. Moderate ECF volume deficit
        a. Apathy
        b. Slow response to questioning, but oriented as to time and place
        c. Cessation of usual activities, such as smoking, chewing gum, reading, or watching television
     2. Severe ECF volume deficit
        a. Reduced tendon reflexes
        b. Stupor
        c. Coma
  B. Gastrointestinal signs
     1. Moderate ECF volume deficit
        Reduced ingestion of food and water
     2. Severe reduction in ECF volume
        a. Nausea and vomiting
        b. Refusal of food and beverages
        c. Silent ileus with tympanites
  C. Cardiovascular signs
     1. Moderate ECF volume deficit
        a. Orthostatic hypotension
        b. Tachycardia with a thready pulse
        c. Slow filling of veins below a venous-occlusion tourniquet
     2. Severe ECF volume deficit
        a. Hypotension even when recumbent
        b. Tachycardia with absent peripheral pulses
        c. Distant heart sounds, with soft A_2
        d. Cold extremities
  D. Signs of reduction in fluid volume in tissues
     1. Moderate ECF volume deficit
        a. Decrease in skin turgor
        b. Longitudinal wrinkling of the tongue

   2. Severe ECF volume deficit
      a. Further decrease in skin turgor
      b. Sunken and soft eyeballs
      c. Atonic muscles
 E. Signs of reduction in energy expenditure
    Fall in body temperature. This occurs if environ-
    mental temperature is less than 85–90 F and if
    there is no infection complicating the illness. An
    ECF volume deficit is the first thing to consider in
    a patient who has decreased body temperature,
    and who has not been unduly chilled by exposure
    to cold environmental temperatures.
Laboratory Findings
   The laboratory findings are of minimal value in diag-
nosing an ECF volume deficit. The findings are listed in
the approximate order of their reliability.
 A. Urine
    [Na^+] and/or [Cl^-] are reduced, usually below 25
    mEq/L and often as low as 1–2 mEq/L. (Excep-
    tions: salt-losing renal disturbances, and ECF vol-
    ume deficit complicated by a severe simple water
    deficit)
 B. Blood
    1. Hematocrit, [Hb], and RBC tend to be above
       normal.
    2. Urea tends to be high.
 C. Plasma
    Protein concentration tends to be above normal.

TREATMENT

   The treatment of an ECF volume deficit is to administer
water containing salt. The tonicity of the fluid and its electrolyte composition must always be chosen in light of the particu-
lar concentration and compositional disturbances that accom-
pany the deficit. For this reason, treatment is detailed in Chapter 7, after compositional disturbances have been discussed.

EXTRACELLULAR FLUID EXCESS

   Extracellular fluid excess is an abnormal water balance state
that is treated only briefly in this book. The most frequent
cause of this condition is heart failure, also known as congestive

failure. A second, less-frequent cause is the nephrotic syndrome. This condition may also occur in Cushing's syndrome.

The specific treatment of ECF volume excess depends upon the cause. In congestive failure, digitalis, diuretics, and low-sodium diets are the sheet anchor of the treatment. These treatments are covered well in most standard medical texts, and the details will not be repeated here.

CLINICAL PICTURE OF ECF VOLUME EXCESS WITHOUT SIGNIFICANT CHANGES IN OSMOLAR CONCENTRATION

History
  A. Dyspnea on exertion or, in more severe cases, at rest
  B. Orthopnea
  C. Paroxysmal nocturnal dyspnea
  D. Rapid weight gain
Physical Examination
  A. Signs of increased ECF volume due to expansion of the plasma volume
    (The plasma volume usually shares in the expanded volume unless there is hypoalbuminemia.)
    1. Elevated venous pressure
    2. Rales at the base of the lungs
    3. Accentuation of pulmonic second sound
    4. Decreased breath sounds. (The involvement of the lungs depends upon the severity and duration of the volume excess.)
  B. Signs of increased ECF volume due to the expansion of the interstitial cell volume
    1. Moderate increase
    Pitting edema in the dependent portion of the body (in the lower extremities of ambulatory patients; in the presacral region of a bedfast patient who is lying on his back)
    2. Severe increase
      a. Anasarca (peritoneal and pleural effusion, with possible pericardial effusion)
      b. Liver palpable if the distention caused by peritoneal fluid is not too great. (The liver is tender if the increase in volume has occurred recently.)

Laboratory Findings

There are no specific findings. SO_4 or inulin space would be increased if measured.

A. Urine

[Na^+] and/or [Cl^-] are above 25 mEq/L.

B. Blood

Hematocrit, [Hb], and RBC tend to be below normal.

C. Plasma

Protein concentration tends to be low.

BIBLIOGRAPHY

Cooke, R. E., and Crowley, L. G.: Replacement of gastric and intestinal fluid losses in surgery, a preliminary report, N. Engl. J. Med. 246:637, 1952.

Dahl, L. K.: Salt intake and salt need, N. Engl. J. Med. 258:1152 and 1205, 1958.

Danowski, T. S., Fergus, E. B., and Mateer, F. M.: The low salt syndromes, Ann. Intern. Med. 43:643, 1955.

Earley, L. E., and Daugharty, T. M.: Sodium metabolism, N. Engl. J. Med. 281:72, 1969.

Goldberger, E.: *A Primer of Water, Electrolyte and Acid-Base Syndromes* (5th ed.; Philadelphia: Lea and Febiger, 1975).

Mahalanabis, D., *et al.*: Oral fluid therapy of cholera among Bangladesh refugees, Johns Hopkins Med. J. 132:197, 1973.

Marriott, H. L.: Water and salt depletion, Br. Med. J. 1:245, 285 and 328, 1947.

Moore, F. D.: Common patterns of water and electrolyte change in injury, surgery and disease, N. Engl. J. Med. 258:277, 325, 377 and 427, 1958.

5 / Acid-Base Disturbances

IN PLASMA AND ECF, the range of pH in normal individuals is quite small. Measured in arterial blood, the range is from 7.36 to 7.42. The pH of venous blood is lower. If venous blood is collected from a limb that has good perfusion, and without use of a tourniquet, the pH will be from 0.04 to 0.05 pH units lower than arterial blood. In disease states, the pH range rarely exceeds 7.00–7.80.

In this chapter, the physiology and diagnosis of the acid-base disturbances will be discussed.

DIAGNOSIS OF ACID-BASE DISTURBANCES

Diagnosis of acid-base states can be made on the basis of the clinical state of the individual, but in this day the clinician relies on the laboratory. The laboratory diagnosis is less subject to error. The clinician should be thoroughly familiar with the characteristic laboratory findings of each disorder. In addition, he must understand the basic physiologic mechanisms that are associated with each of the disease states.

For the evaluation of an acid-base disorder, there is general agreement that one should obtain a laboratory determination of these three values:
1. Blood or plasma P_{CO_2}
2. Blood or plasma pH
3. A measure of the change in plasma bicarbonate. This may be reported in various ways. Common ways are as calculated $[HCO_3^-]_p$, CO_2 content, delta base, and buffer base.

These values are best determined from arterial blood. Commonly, the P_{CO_2} and pH are determined directly, and the third value is calculated from these two by using the Henderson-Hasselbalch equation.

BUFFERS

A buffer is a solution of a weak acid and its salt. The acid and salt are called a buffer pair. The buffer resists a marked change in concentration of H^+ when either strong acids or strong bases are added to the solution.

PLASMA BUFFERS

The buffer pairs in plasma, with their appropriate total millimolar concentrations, are:

$$\frac{NaHCO_3}{H_2CO_3} \;\; 27 \text{ mM} \qquad \frac{Na_2HPO_4}{NaH_2PO_4} \;\; 2 \text{ mM} \qquad \frac{Na \text{ protein}}{H \text{ protein}} \;\; 16 \text{ mM}$$

The ratio of each pair and the pH of the solution are related by the Henderson-Hasselbalch equation, which states:

$$pH = pK + \log\frac{base}{acid}$$

In the equation, base is the molar concentration of the salt in the pair, and acid is the molar concentration of the acid. The functional pK of the bicarbonate system is 6.1; the pK of the phosphate system is 6.8 in body fluids. The various proteins each have different pK values, and it is not practical to express a pK for the mixed proteins of plasma.

It is important to understand these concepts:

1. The Henderson-Hasselbalch equation states that the pH and the ratio of buffers is such that the pH (the negative log of $[H^+]$) cannot be changed without changing the ratio.
2. It is axiomatic that there cannot be two different $[H^+]$ at a given place in a solution at the same time.
3. It then follows, if there is more than one buffer system in a solution, when the pH changes, the ratio of all the systems will change. In so doing, all buffer systems contribute to the buffering of the pH change.
4. A corollary to the first three statements is that only the status of one buffer pair in a disease state is needed. If the changes in one buffer pair are known, this is sufficient information to know what is happening to the other buffer pairs.

The bicarbonate system is chosen for use in diagnosis and treatment of disease states. It is chosen because:

1. In plasma and ECF it is in the highest molar concentration, and therefore it is the more effective buffer.

2. The acid H_2CO_3 is not a fixed acid. The body can decrease $[H_2CO_3]_p$ by the reaction

$$H_2CO_3 \rightarrow H_2O + CO_2$$

The CO_2 is blown off by the lung. If necessary, the body can increase $[H_2CO_3]$ by slowing ventilation, retaining CO_2, and thus shifting this reaction to the left.

CHLORIDE SHIFT

In addition to the buffers of plasma, the hemoglobin of the red cells buffers the change in pH of the plasma. It does so by the chloride shift shown in Figure 5-1.

As a result of the lowering of P_{CO_2} and the elevation of P_{O_2}, the following changes occur:

1. The $[HCO_3^-]$ of plasma and erythrocytes decreases.
2. The Cl^- content of the erythrocytes decreases.
3. The $[Cl^-]$ of plasma increases.
4. The total fixed cation content of the erythrocytes does not change.
5. The water content and volume of the erythrocytes decrease.

These changes occur in the reverse direction in the capillaries of the tissues.

The changes in bicarbonate content occur whether or not there is a change in P_{O_2} in the plasma. For example, the P_{CO_2} might be markedly decreased by hyperventilation, with little change in P_{O_2}, but still there would be a marked change in plasma bicarbonate concentration.

In addition to the change in $[HCO_3^-]_p$ due to the chloride shift, a decrease in P_{CO_2} produces a decrease in $[HCO_3^-]_p$ by these reactions between the plasma buffer systems:

$$NaHCO_3 + NaH_2PO_4 \rightarrow Na_2HPO_4 + H_2CO_3$$
$$NaHCO_3 + H \text{ protein} \rightarrow Na \text{ protein} + H_2CO_3$$

The H_2CO_3 formed in each case can decompose to H_2O and CO_2.

These reactions between the plasma buffer systems account for 20-25% of the change in bicarbonate concentration that occurs in the plasma of whole blood.

Of course, if the P_{CO_2} is increased, the plasma bicarbonate

Chloride Shift
In capillaries of lungs

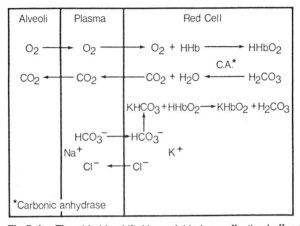

Fig 5–1.—The chloride shift. Hemoglobin is an effective buffer of the pH of plasma as shown through this series of reactions. In the capillaries of the lungs, as the P_{CO_2} is lowered, hemoglobin prevents a marked alkaline change in the pH of plasma by reducing the $[HCO_3^-]$ of the bicarbonate-carbonic acid buffer pair in the plasma. (The quantitation of this effect is shown in Fig 5–2.) All reactions are in response to changes in concentrations of the reactants. The reactions are reversed in the capillaries of the tissues when P_{CO_2} rises and P_{O_2} falls.

increases by the reverse of the reaction just shown, in addition to the chloride shift.

The quantitative effect of merely changing P_{CO_2} on the $[HCO_3^-]_p$ in whole blood with 15 gm/100 ml hemoglobin is shown in Figure 5–2. This is the normal buffer slope. If the hemoglobin concentration were less, the slope of the line would be more nearly horizontal.

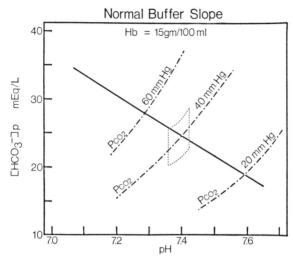

Fig 5–2.—The normal buffer slope. This shows the change in $[HCO_3^-]_p$ that occurs in whole blood with a change in plasma pH produced by a change in Pco_2. The change in bicarbonate is primarily due to the chloride shift. The slope of the line would be different for a different Hb concentration.,

ABNORMAL ACID-BASE STATES

The following general principles apply to all the basic disturbances in acid-base balance. Read them, and then try to understand them in terms of each example that follows.

1. The primary disturbance in acid-base balance may manifest itself as an increase or decrease in either the numerator or denominator of the buffer pair. In the bicarbonate-carbonic acid system then there are four primary disturbances to consider:
   a. Concentration of H_2CO_3 increases
   b. Concentration of H_2CO_3 decreases
   c. Concentration of $NaHCO_3$ increases
   d. Concentration of $NaHCO_3$ decreases
2. In a disease state, the primary disturbance usually persists for some time because the body cannot quickly revert the

disturbance back to normal. (For example, if CO_2 is retained because of a severe pneumonia, the PCO_2 will rise and remain high until the person recovers from the pneumonia.)

3. The primary disturbance changes the pH away from normal. The body can ameliorate this disturbance by introducing a *compensatory* change in the *other* member of the buffer pair so that the ratio of the pair is more nearly normal. This then makes the $[H^+]$ of plasma and ECF more nearly normal.

The manner in which the chloride shift and the bicarbonate buffer system interact in each disturbance will be given for an idealized case.

METABOLIC ACIDOSIS

ETIOLOGY

1. Loss of bicarbonate may occur through buffering of strong acids. The classic example of this is diabetic acidosis. However, lactic acid may be produced in excess, or strong acids may be retained by the kidney in renal disease. Starvation also leads to excessive production of strong acids.
2. Loss of bicarbonate may occur directly as the result of loss of any body fluid which contains HCO_3^- in a concentration that is higher than plasma. This may happen in biliary fistulas, pancreatic fistulas, diarrhea, or occasionally in vomiting of duodenal contents.
3. In certain renal diseases there may be excessive and inappropriate loss of bicarbonate. In chronic renal disease, there is retention of fixed acids.

The following discussion refers to Figure 5–3.

UNCOMPENSATED STATE (POINT B)

1. Accumulation of strong acids which react with $NaHCO_3$ in plasma produce carbonic acid which decomposes to CO_2 and H_2O.
2. The respiratory system blows off the extra CO_2 formed and thereby keeps PCO_2 constant.
3. $[HCO_3^-]_p$ decreases.
4. pH of plasma becomes more acid.

In the example, the $[HCO_3^-]_p$ fell from 24.5 to 15.0 mEq/L. It is assumed that the PCO_2 remained constant. In some cases of acidosis, the rate of production of H_2CO_3 from the reaction between the acid and bicarbonate might be so fast that the respiratory system could not keep pace with the production, and PCO_2 might rise transiently. The line shown, A-B, is the PCO_2 40 mm Hg isobar.

COMPENSATION (LINE B-C)

1. It is assumed that the excessive rate of production of the strong acid ceases.
2. The respiratory center is stimulated by the acidosis to lower the PCO_2.
3. The chloride shift further lowers $[HCO_3^-]_p$.
4. Plasma pH rises toward normal.

This idealized case is assumed to be a diabetic who is given insulin to slow the rate of production of the keto acids. Normally he would receive other treatment, but for this example it is assumed that he does not. The stimulation of the respiratory center involves the interrelationships between plasma and cerebrospinal fluid PCO_2 and $[HCO_3^-]$ which are not detailed in this book. The mechanism is responsible for a lag in the respiratory system's response to the acidosis. It takes about 12 hours to achieve maximum compensation.

As the PCO_2 is lowered, there is a further lowering of $[HCO_3^-]_p$ to 11 mEq/L. However, the net result is a rise in the plasma pH to 7.33. The line B-C is approximately parallel to the normal buffer slope of plasma.

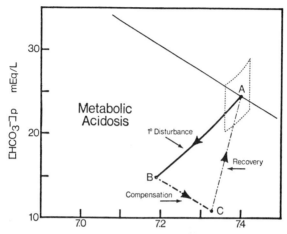

Fig 5–3.—The change in plasma pH and $[HCO_3^-]_p$ in metabolic acidosis. This shows an idealized case with changes during the primary disturbance, compensation, and recovery.

RECOVERY (LINE C-A)

1. If the metabolic acidosis is due to chronic renal disease and retention of strong acids, spontaneous recovery will not occur.
2. If metabolic acidosis is due to other etiologies, recovery will probably occur with adequate treatment.
3. The kidney will produce an acid urine, and thereby produce bicarbonate which is returned to the ECF.
4. $[HCO_3^-]_p$ will gradually increase and return to normal.
5. P_{CO_2} will gradually return to normal.
6. Plasma pH will return to normal.

The kidney will excrete an acid urine, with pH about 4.5–5.0. It will contain a high concentration of NH_4^+ and have a high titratable acidity. In producing such a urine, the kidney exchanges Na^+ in the urine for H^+ from carbonic acid in the renal tubular cell. The $NaHCO_3$ formed in the cell is then reabsorbed into the ECF. If the process is unassisted by specific replacement therapy, it will take several days to return the plasma $[HCO_3^-]$ to normal. An adjunct to this renal mechanism is the metabolism of the excess organic acids in the ECF. As they are metabolized, they are replaced by bicarbonate.

METABOLIC ALKALOSIS

ETIOLOGY

The plasma bicarbonate must be primarily elevated. This may be brought about by:

1. Ingestion or infusion of $NaHCO_3$
2. Inappropriate retention of bicarbonate by the kidney, which often occurs in potassium deficit
3. Vomiting, in a person who produces HCl in stomach secretions

In the process of formation of HCl by the stomach, $NaHCO_3$ is returned to the ECF. The HCl produced in response to one meal causes little change in $[HCO_3^-]_p$. The change is transient because the HCl is, in effect, reabsorbed and the process is reversed. If there is persistent vomiting, there is a net loss of HCl and a metabolic alkalosis results.

The following discussion refers to Figure 5–4.

UNCOMPENSATED STATE (POINT B)

1. Plasma bicarbonate is elevated because of ingestion of $NaHCO_3$ (or other factors just noted).
2. Respiratory system maintains normal Pco_2.
3. Plasma pH becomes alkaline.
4. Kidney begins excretion of $NaHCO_3$ promptly so urine pH reaches maximum alkalinity of 7.0–7.5. (This is not true in K^+ deficiency, where the kidney is the cause of the alkalosis.)

Again, as in metabolic acidosis, the respiratory system at first will tend to maintain the normal Pco_2. This is due to the interrelationships of plasma and cerebrospinal fluid Pco_2 and $[HCO_3^-]$. In the example, plasma bicarbonate rose to 40 mEq/L, giving a pH of 7.61.

COMPENSATION (LINE B-C)

1. Ventilation is decreased so the Pco_2 rises.
2. The chloride shift causes a further rise in $[HCO_3^-]_p$.
3. Plasma pH falls.

The respiratory compensation takes place over a period of about 12 hours. In the example, the $[HCO_3^-]_p$ rose further, from 40 to 45 mEq/L. However the rise in Pco_2 was sufficient to lower the HCO_3^- to H_2CO_3 ratio so that the pH returned toward normal.

RECOVERY (LINE C-A)

1. The kidney excretes HCO_3^-. The urine remains alkaline during this process.
2. The respiratory system gradually lowers Pco_2.
3. The plasma pH returns to normal.

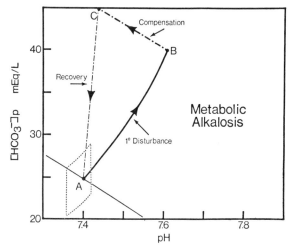

Fig 5–4.—The change in plasma pH and $[HCO_3^-]_p$ in metabolic alkalosis. This shows an idealized case with changes during the primary disturbance, compensation, and recovery.

RESPIRATORY ALKALOSIS

ETIOLOGY

Something must happen to cause the individual to excrete CO_2 at a rate greater than it is produced. This lowers PCO_2. The respiratory center may be stimulated abnormally and directly, as in encephalitis. It may be stimulated reflexly, for example, when hypoxia drives respiration. Or the respiratory center may be stimulated from cortical centers, for example, when hyperventilation occurs with an anxiety state.

The following discussion refers to Figure 5–5.

UNCOMPENSATED STATE (POINT B)

1. Excess excretion of CO_2 lowers $[H_2CO_3]$ and PCO_2.
2. The chloride shift lowers $[HCO_3^-]_p$.
3. The pH of plasma becomes more alkaline.

In the example, the excretion of CO_2 lowers PCO_2 from 40 to 20 mm Hg. The values move along the normal buffer slope to point B. The pH is 7.60 and the $[HCO_3^-]_p$ is 19.0 mEq/L. These changes take place immediately with the hyperventilation.

COMPENSATION (LINE B-C)

1. Urine becomes more alkaline as the kidney excretes HCO_3^-.
2. $[HCO_3^-]_p$ falls slowly. Maximum compensation is achieved in about 2–3 days.
3. pH of plasma becomes more nearly normal.

In the example, the kidney lowered the $[HCO_3^-]_p$ from 19.0 to 13.0 mEq/L. The values move along a line which is the PCO_2 20 mm Hg isobar. If the kidney is normal, the urine pH will be near maximum alkalinity (7.0–7.5). The excretion of bicarbonate in the urine begins promptly but the amount excreted does not lower the plasma bicarbonate rapidly, so that the process takes 2–3 days to reach maximum compensation. In mild cases, compensation might be reached sooner.

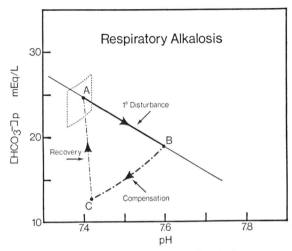

Fig 5–5.—The change in plasma pH and $[HCO_3^-]_p$ in respiratory alkalosis. This shows an idealized case with changes during the primary disturbance, compensation, and recovery.

RECOVERY (LINE C-A)

Recovery of respiratory alkalosis will usually occur. The ventilatory defect reverses itself and the P_{CO_2} rises back to normal. The kidney slowly changes the $[HCO_3^-]_p$ back to normal.

RESPIRATORY ACIDOSIS

ETIOLOGY

The concentration of H_2CO_3 increases because of the retention of CO_2 that is caused by some impairment in pulmonary function. This could be due to:

1. Poor exchange of CO_2 across an alveolar membrane when it is thickened.
2. Inadequate ventilation.
3. Increased CO_2 concentration of inspired air. (This is not commonly encountered.)

The following discussion refers to Figure 5–6.

UNCOMPENSATED STATE (POINT B)

1. Retention of CO_2 raises $[H_2CO_3]_p$ and P_{CO_2}.
2. The chloride shift raises $[HCO_3^-]_p$.
3. The pH of plasma becomes more acid.

In the example, the retention of CO_2 raises P_{CO_2} from 40 to 60 mm Hg. The values move along the normal buffer slope to point B. The pH is 7.28 and $[HCO_3^-]_p$ is 28 mEq/L. These changes take place immediately.

COMPENSATION (LINE B-C)

1. The urine becomes more acid with the kidney retaining HCO_3^-.
2. $[HCO_3^-]_p$ rises slowly. Maximum compensation is achieved in about 2–3 days.
3. pH of plasma becomes more nearly normal.

In the example, the kidney increased the $[HCO_3^-]_p$ from 28 to 32 mEq/L. The P_{CO_2} remained at 60 mm Hg. (This assumes that the problem causing the acidosis is not changing.) The change in $[HCO_3^-]$ changes the ratio of the buffer pair so that the pH of plasma then shifts toward normal. If the kidney is normal, the urine pH should be near maximum acidity (4.5–5.0). The retention of HCO_3^- by the kidney begins promptly, but the amount retained per unit time does not raise bicarbonate rapidly, so that the process takes 2–3 days to reach

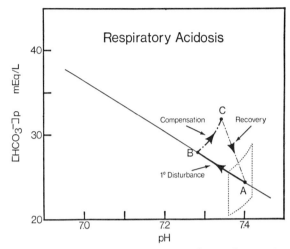

Fig 5–6.—The change in plasma pH and $[HCO_3^-]_p$ in respiratory acidosis. This shows an idealized case with changes during the primary disturbance, compensation, and recovery.

maximum compensation. In milder cases of acidosis, maximum compensation might be reached sooner.

RECOVERY (LINE C-A)

1. If the pulmonary defect is reversible, as in a pneumonia, then recovery can occur.
2. If the pulmonary defect is not reversible, as in chronic emphysema, then recovery cannot occur, and the patient will live the rest of his life in a state of compensated respiratory acidosis.
3. When recovery occurs, usually the P_{CO_2} is lowered slowly, and the kidney slowly changes the $[HCO_3^-]_p$ so that the values move along the line, as indicated, and return to normal.

An infrequent, but important, exception to this course of the disease should be known to all physicians. A foreign body may obstruct the respiratory tree, and impair CO_2 excretion. If the foreign body is removed within a few hours, no problem is encountered. However, if the obstruction persists for 1 or 2 days or longer, then compensation takes place with the elevated $[HCO_3^-]_p$. If the foreign body is now removed the P_{CO_2} usually quickly returns to normal, leaving the individual with a metabolic alkalosis. The alkalosis may depress respiration even to the point of death.

In such cases, the physician must be alert that this can happen. He must devise some treatment to allow the P_{CO_2} to slowly return to normal, so the kidney can lower the $[HCO_3^-]_p$ to normal gradually. A simple procedure would be to have the patient partially rebreathe his own CO_2 by artificially enlarging his respiratory dead space.

DEFINITION OF DELTA BASE

Delta base is the vertical displacement of a point from the buffer slope. It is a positive value if the point is above the line and a negative value if it is below the line. Another acceptable terminology is Base Excess and Base Deficit for the positive and negative values of delta base, respectively.

The advantages of this calculation are that they separate the change in $[HCO_3^-]_p$ due to the chloride shift from the change due to other buffering and compensatory mechanisms. This is demonstrated by considering the example in Figure 5–6. Point B represents a $[HCO_3^-]_p$ of 28 mEq/L, which is an increase in $[HCO_3^-]_p$. But this increase is all due to the buffering effect of Hb through the chloride shift. The delta base is zero, and this tells the clinician that there has been no renal compensation at this point. When the conditions move from point B to point C, the $[HCO_3^-]_p$ is now 32 mEq/L. The combined increase and movement of the point to the right give a vertical displacement of 6 mEq/L. Point C then indicates a delta base of plus 6 mEq/L.

LIMITATIONS OF THE CALCULATION OF DELTA BASE

The examples of acid-base disturbances given in the first part of this chapter are plotted on the normal buffer slope which is determined on whole blood in vitro. There are two things which alter this buffer slope in vivo. First, as the $[HCO_3^-]_p$ rises or falls, the change in concentration in plasma is ameliorated by the new concentration coming to a steady state with respect to the $[HCO_3^-]$ in interstitial fluids. This tends to decrease the slope of the line.

This effect is offset by the second factor. There is a buffering of the change in $[H^+]$ of interstitial fluid by an appropriate exchange of Cl^- for HCO_3^- across the plasma membrane of skeletal muscle cells and other cells in the body. The HCO_3^- comes out of the cells in acidosis, and enters the cells in alkalosis. The result of the buffering is to make the line of the buffer slope steeper. Attempts have been made to measure directly the buffer slope line in vivo. Such studies indicate that, although the two effects tend to cancel each other, the slope in vivo often varies from that of the blood in vitro. The degree and direction of variation is not predictable. However, the in-vitro line is usually a reasonable approximation of the line observed in vivo.

It follows that the buffer slope line for whole blood of two individuals with identical [Hb] would be the same, but that the in-vivo buffer slope line might be quite different because of differences in either tissue-buffering capabilities, or in the ratio of plasma volume to interstitial cell volume. It is important for the clinician to remember these variations and to realize that a calculation of delta base for a patient is subject to these errors.

The characteristic changes in laboratory values that are associated with each type of acid-base disturbance are shown in Table 5–1.

TABLE 5–1.—THE LABORATORY CHARACTERISTICS OF ACID-BASE STATES

STATE	PLASMA pH	P_{CO_2} MM HG	$[HCO_3^-]_p$ mEQ/L	DELTA BASE mEQ/L
Normal*	7.36–7.42	36–46	22–26	−2.5 to +2.5
Respiratory acidosis, uncompensated	Low	High	Normal	Normal
Respiratory acidosis, compensated	Low normal or slightly low	High	High	Positive value >2.5
Respiratory alkalosis, uncompensated	High	Low	Normal	Normal
Respiratory alkalosis, compensated	High normal or slightly high	Low	Low	Negative value >2.5
Metabolic acidosis, uncompensated	Low	Normal	Low	Negative value >2.5
Metabolic acidosis, compensated	Low normal or slightly low	Low	Low	Negative value >2.5
Metabolic alkalosis, uncompensated	High	Normal	High	Positive value >2.5
Metabolic alkalosis, compensated	High normal or slightly high	High	High	Positive value >2.5

*Normal values are for arterial blood plasma.

EXTRAVASCULAR BUFFERING

In addition to the buffering by the chloride shift and plasma buffers, it is now evident from the work in Pitts' laboratory that there is considerable buffering of the ECF by other mechanisms. These changes are briefly summarized here. Of the changes, the movement of K^+ into and out of the ECF with changes in pH is probably of the most importance clinically.

METABOLIC ACIDOSIS

In severe acidosis, a little over half of the acid is buffered in some other manner than by red cells and plasma. Hydrogen ions leave the ECF in exchange for both Na^+ and K^+. The exchange for K^+ represents about 15% of the total buffering, and the exchange for Na^+ about 36%. This exchange is thought to be across cell membranes, although exchange with Na^+ in bone cannot be ruled out.

METABOLIC ALKALOSIS

With an excess intake of bicarbonate, 67% of the bicarbonate remains in the ECF. Most of the remainder is buffered by H^+ moving out of cells in exchange for Na^+. A small amount of bicarbonate is converted to H_2CO_3 by the production of lactic acid. The H_2CO_3 is then dissociated to CO_2 and H_2O, and the CO_2 blown off by the lung. More recent work indicates that K^+ also moves into cells in metabolic alkalosis.

RESPIRATORY ALKALOSIS

In respiratory alkalosis, the plasma bicarbonate is lowered by other mechanisms in addition to renal compensation. These mechanisms are more effective than renal compensation in the early phase of the disturbance. As already indicated, the bicarbonate can be lowered by the chloride shift. However, it can be further lowered by approximately the same amount by an increase in the production of lactic acid. Another means of reduction is by exchange of Na^+ and K^+ in ECF for intracellular H^+. The exchange for Na^+ is about four times the exchange for K^+, and the two combined represent one-fifth of the total buffering in an animal without kidneys.

RESPIRATORY ACIDOSIS

Similarly, the increase in PCO_2 in respiratory acidosis is buffered by a rise in bicarbonate concentration due to other factors than renal compensation. About 33% of the rise by these other mechanisms is accounted for by the chloride shift. Approximately 15% is brought about by the exchange of ECF H^+ for intracellular K^+. This tends to raise the ECF $[K^+]$, but if renal function is normal, the K^+ will be excreted. A small amount of the increase in $[HCO_3^-]_p$ is brought about by a reduction in the organic acid content of plasma. There is a further rise in $[HCO_3^-]_p$ that is thought to be caused by cellular mechanisms, but the exact nature of the mechanism is not known.

ANION GAP

In normal plasma the sum of the concentrations of Cl^- plus HCO_3^- is 130 mEq/L. This is 12 mEq/L less than the normal Na^+ concentration and is 17 mEq/L less than the normal Na^+ plus K^+ concentration. Either of these differences has been called the "anion gap." If the K^+ concentration is abnormal, the second calculation is the better one. Any increase in the anion gap is most likely due to an increase in the total concentration of organic acids in plasma.

Increases in organic acids occur in diabetic acidosis, lactic acidosis, and in certain types of poisoning. The observation that the "gap" has increased is often the first clue to the increase in the organic acids, and should lead to an investigation for the cause of the large gap.

LACTIC ACIDOSIS

Lactic acidosis is one mechanism of production of a metabolic acidosis. Normal lactic acid blood levels are 0.5–1.5 mEq/L. Pyruvic acid levels are 0.05–0.15 mEq/L. When both acid concentrations are elevated proportionately so that the ratio of lactic to pyruvic acid is relatively constant, such elevations are less serious than when the lactic acid is elevated out of proportion to the pyruvic acid levels. Lactic acidemia is commonly stated to exist when the lactic acid concentration is above 7.0 mEq/L.

Lactic acidosis is usually secondary to tissue hypoxia. It occurs transiently in strenuous exercise, and this is not serious. It may occur in any disease state in which there is circulatory insufficiency, such as in surgical shock due to hypovolemia, or in acute myocardial infarction with reduced arterial blood pressure. This is known as secondary lactic acidemia. Although this may represent a process associated with a moribund state, it still should be treated vigorously as outlined next.

Increased lactic acid may occur in association with a respiratory alkalosis with blood concentrations as high as 15–20 mEq/L. This production of lactic acid serves as a compensatory mechanism. The plasma pH will be high. Treatment should be directed at the cause of the respiratory alkalosis. In these cases administration of sodium bicarbonate would be contraindicated.

Less frequent in occurrence is the condition of idiopathic, or primary, lactic acidosis. This is characterized by a sudden increase in lactic acid concentration without apparent tissue hypoxia.

Either primary or secondary lactic acidosis is associated with dyspnea and tachypnea, usually of the Kussmaul type. There is stupor or coma and, characteristically, the onset is sudden.

The prognosis in either primary or secondary lactic acidosis is grave. If tissue hypoxia exists, treatment should be directed both toward relieving the tissue hypoxia and administering $NaHCO_3$ solutions to relieve the acidosis. Sodium lactate solutions would not be useful in treatment since the plasma lactic acid level is already elevated.

Treatment of primary lactic acidosis is unsatisfactory. It has been likened to the treatment of diabetic acidosis in the pre-insulin days. Until a better understanding exists of a more basic defect in the metabolism in this disease, it is doubtful that treatment will be adequate. At present, the best treatment is to administer $NaHCO_3$ or THAM (tromethamine) solutions in large doses. Treatment should be vigorous in an attempt to prevent lethal reductions in plasma pH.

TREATMENT OF ACID-BASE DISTURBANCES

ACIDOSIS OF DILUTION

The principle of "the acidosis of dilution" is important in understanding the treatment of any acid-base condition. Stated simply, the administration of an isotonic salt solution which contains chloride as the only anion will dilute the bicarbonate concentration of the ECF. The Pco_2 and, hence, the H_2CO_3 concentration is set by the respiratory system. Although theoretically the H_2CO_3 would be diluted by the fluid, in fact the respiratory system retains sufficient metabolic CO_2 to maintain the acid-half of the buffer pair at a constant concentration. As a result, in a normal individual a metabolic acidosis is produced by the dilution effect. The severity of the acidosis depends upon the ratio of the initial volume of the ECF and the volume of the salt solution that is administered.

An acidosis of dilution is illustrated by the following example. Consider a patient with an ECF volume reduced from 14 to 12 liters. The $[HCO_3^-]_p$ is normal, 27 mEq/L. If the saltwater loss is replaced with 2 liters of 0.9% NaCl, the calculations would be:

	ECF volume (liters)		$[HCO_3^-]$ (mEq/L)		Total HCO_3^- (mEq)
Initial status of ECF	12	×	27	=	324
Add	2	×	0	=	0
Resulting in	14	×	$[HCO_3^-]_{at}$ =		324

where $[HCO_3^-]_{at}$ is the bicarbonate concentration of the ECF after treatment. Calculating, this would be 23.1 mEq/L. This would be a delta base of minus 3.9 mEq/L. The patient is in a mild metabolic acidosis as a result of the dilution of the bicarbonate.

In a normal individual, the kidney would correct this acidosis rather promptly. In the treatment of a patient with a combined ECF deficit and a metabolic acidosis, it would be important to avoid further dilution of the $[HCO_3^-]$ in treating the saltwater deficit. Also, if the ECF deficit were severe but not complicated by an acidosis, treatment with solutions which had only Cl^- as the anion would induce a moderately severe metabolic acidosis. This dilution would be produced by administering either 0.9% NaCl, or Ringer's solution.

PREVENTION OF ACIDOSIS OF DILUTION

Lactated Ringer's solution contains 27 mEq/L sodium lactate. The lactate is metabolized and $NaHCO_3$ is produced. In severe liver disease, the rate of lactate metabolism may be severely reduced; therefore, sodium lactate solutions should be given with caution.

Bicarbonate cannot be mixed with Ringer's solution because the calcium would be precipitated as calcium carbonate. A sodium bicarbonate-sodium chloride mixture in solution could be given to prevent the acidosis of dilution, but such a solution is not in general use.

METABOLIC ACIDOSIS

If the acidosis is complicated by an ECF deficit, the choices of treatment are:
1. Lactated Ringer's solution. In mild acidosis, this is probably adequate. It does not markedly raise the bicarbonate concentration.
2. 1/6 M sodium lactate. This will rapidly increase the bicarbonate concentration of the ECF. It should be used in severe acidosis. In addition, the patient will need some solution containing Cl^-.
3. Isotonic $NaHCO_3$ solution. The same comments as in choice 2 apply here.

If the acidosis is not complicated by an appreciable ECF volume deficit, i.e., if volume is normal or increased, the choices of treatment are:
1. Only 1/6 M sodium lactate, or
2. Only isotonic $NaHCO_3$ solution, or
3. Only adequate 5% glucose in water to replace insensible loss and insure adequate urine output; let the kidney correct the acidosis.

METABOLIC ALKALOSIS

If the alkalosis is complicated by an ECF volume deficit, the choices of treatment are:
1. In mild cases, 0.9% NaCl or Ringer's solution. The acidosis of dilution would now be helpful in correcting the high $[HCO_3^-]_p$.

2. In severe cases, 1/6 M NH_4Cl given intravenously. The rate of administration should not exceed 1 liter in 3 hours. At higher rates, the elevation of $[NH_4^+]_p$ may cause CNS symptoms of confusion and disorientation. Since NH_4^+ is converted to urea in the liver, this solution should not be given in cases of liver disease because ammonium toxicity may result.

3. NH_4Cl given by mouth in a daily dose of 6–12 gm. Enteric-coated tablets are absorbed slowly, so that uncoated tablets should be considered even though they may cause gastric irritation.

4. HCl administered by mouth. Five milliliters of 10% HCl in a full glass of water can be drunk through a glass straw to avoid damage to the teeth. If this is repeated 4 times daily, it represents 56 mEq/day of acid administered, which is the equivalent of about 3 gm of NH_4Cl.

In addition, in choices 2 through 4 some sodium chloride solution would be needed to correct the saltwater deficit. This could be given as 0.9% NaCl, or as Ringer's solution.

If no ECF deficit exists, the same principles apply, except that no extra sodium chloride need be administered.

RESPIRATORY ACIDOSIS

The primary disturbance of respiratory acidosis is a respiratory problem. The specifics of therapy are not covered in this book. It must be remembered that the primary cause might be completely reversed by specific treatment, as in an acute pneumonia. On the other hand, complete reversal of the process may not be possible, as in a case of far-advanced pulmonary emphysema, or pulmonary fibrosis.

In a case of respiratory acidosis with no saltwater loss, the only fluids needed would be water by mouth, or 5% glucose in water intravenously, to replace insensible loss and allow adequate fluid for urine production. The principles of treating acid-base balance become important when respiratory acidosis is associated with saltwater loss. Under these circumstances, it is important to avoid the acidosis of dilution. If the respiratory acidosis were uncompensated, diluting the $[HCO_3^-]_p$ would lower the pH even further, and the kidney would have to retain even more HCO_3^- to accomplish compensation than it otherwise would, had the error in treatment not been made.

If the respiratory acidosis were compensated, then diluting the high $[HCO_3^-]_p$ would take away the benefits of the compensation. When salt water is needed in a respiratory acidosis, then a lactated Ringer's solution should be given. Such a solution will generate 27 mEq/L HCO_3^-; even this will cause some dilution of a higher bicarbonate concentration in the ECF. In most cases, the load placed on the kidney would be minor and the kidney would be able to make the fine adjustments in the $[HCO_3^-]_p$ after the fluid was administered.

RESPIRATORY ALKALOSIS

The primary disturbance of respiratory alkalosis is not necessarily a respiratory problem. Quite often the alkalosis is secondary to a hyperventilation caused by an anemic hypoxia. The underlying condition must be carefully evaluated and treated.

If the respiratory alkalosis is complicated by a saltwater deficit, then it is possible that the salt water will be needed before the alkalosis can be reversed. This might occur, for example, in a patient at high altitude with hypoxic hypoxia causing the hyperventilation, and with saltwater loss due to diarrhea.

Clinical judgment plays an important part in the treatment of a given case. If the alkalosis were uncompensated, then administering even a lactated Ringer's solution would add more bicarbonate for the kidney to excrete in order to achieve compensation. If the alkalosis is compensated, then it is important not to give high concentrations of sodium lactate or of sodium bicarbonate because these would reverse the compensation.

If large volumes of salt water are needed in such a case, isotonic NaCl could be alternated with lactated Ringer's solution in order to avoid either a marked dilution of the HCO_3^- that is present, or a marked elevation of it.

OTHER SYSTEMS OF GRAPHING ACID-BASE DISTURBANCES

The diagrams presented in this chapter are not the only way in which the concepts of acid-base can be graphed. The objective of all diagrams is to aid the clinician in easily separating the metabolic and respiratory components of acid-base disturbances. Almost all of the methods of diagramming use values that are related to the Henderson-Hasselbalch equation. Each method has its own advantage. The value of a given method depends primarily upon the individual clinician's familiarity with that system of presentation.

The diagram used here was developed by Davenport. Other diagrams that are frequently used, together with their developers, are:

1. A plot of pH and log P_{CO_2}. (Astrup)
2. A plot of buffer base and P_{CO_2}. (Singer)
3. A plot of log P_{CO_2} and log CO_2 content. (Peters and Van Slyke)
4. A plot of pH and log P_{CO_2}. (Siggaard-Anderson)
5. A diagram of standard bicarbonate. (Jergensen and Astrup)

BIBLIOGRAPHY

Astrup, P.: A new approach to acid-base metabolism, Clin. Chem. 7:1, 1961.

Davenport, H. W.: *The ABC of Acid-Base Chemistry* (5th ed.; Chicago: University of Chicago Press, 1969).

Eichenholz, A., Mulhausen, R. O., and Blumentals, A.: Management of metabolic alkalosis in patients with azotemia; a study of 42 patients, Arch. Intern. Med. 114:236, 1964.

Goldberger, E.: *A Primer of Water, Electrolyte and Acid-Base Syndromes* (5th ed.; Philadelphia: Lea and Febiger, 1975).

Huckabee, W. E.: Hyperlactatemia, Helv. Med. Acta, 35:363, 1970.

Levitin, H.: Acid-Base Balance, in Bondy, P. K. (ed.): *Duncan's Diseases of Metabolism* (6th ed.; Philadelphia: W. B. Saunders, 1969).

Nahas, G. G.: Current concepts of acid-base measurements, Ann. N.Y. Acad. Sci., 133:1, 1966.

Phillipson, E. A., and Sproule, B. J.: The clinical significance of elevated blood lactate, Can. Med. Assoc. J. 92:1334, 1965.

Pitts, R. F.: *Physiology of the Kidney and Body Fluids* (3d ed.; Chicago: Year Book Medical Publishers, 1974).

Relman, A. S.: The acidosis of renal disease, Am. J. Med. 44:706, 1968.

Schwartz, W. B.: Defense of extracellular pH during acute and chronic hypercapnia, Ann. N.Y. Acad. Sci. 133:125, 1966.

Shires, G. T., and Holman, J.: Dilution acidosis, Ann. Intern. Med. 28:557, 1948.

Singer, R. B.: A new diagram for the visualization and interpretation of acid-base changes, Am. J. Med. Sci. 221:199, 1951.

Tranquada, R. E., Grant, W. J., and Peterson, C. R.: Lactic acidosis, Arch. Intern. Med. 117:192, 1966.

Van Slyke, D. D., and Sendroy, J., Jr.: Studies of gas and electrolyte equilibria in blood. XV. Line charts for graphic calculations by the Henderson-Hasselbalch equation and for calculating plasma carbon dioxide content from whole blood content, J. Biol. Chem. 79:781, 1928.

Waters, W. C., III, Hall, J. D., and Schwartz, W. B.: Spontaneous lactic acidosis. The nature of the acid-base disturbance and considerations in diagnosis and management, Am. J. Med. 35:781, 1963.

Winters, R. W., Engel, K., and Dell, R. B.: *Acid-Base Physiology in Medicine* (2d ed.; Cleveland: The London Co., 1969).

6 / K$^+$ and Mg^{++} Disturbances

POTASSIUM AND MAGNESIUM are present in high concentrations in cells, and low concentrations in ECF. In each case, excesses or deficits of total body content are estimated by determining plasma or serum levels, and these determinations do not truly reflect the excess or deficit of the ion in question in the body.

BASIC PHYSIOLOGY OF POTASSIUM

The understanding of the management of a patient's potassium balance is derived from the following basic facts:
1. There is K$^+$ present in all natural foods, and most prepared foods. Sugar and purified fats and oils are the principal potassium-free foods.
2. There is K$^+$ in all body fluids. The kidney can excrete urine with high $[K^+]$. In K$^+$ deficiency, the kidney cannot produce urine that is virtually free of K$^+$, so there is continued loss by this route. Secretions of the stomach have $[K^+]$ greater than ECF, usually 15–20 mEq/L. Other body fluids have $[K^+]$ about the same as that of plasma. Reasonable normal values are given in Table 6–1.

TABLE 6–1.—$[K^+]$ OF VARIOUS BODY FLUIDS

FLUID	$[K^+]$ MEQ/L
Plasma	3.5–5.5
Sweat	5–10
Saliva	14–26
Total gastric juice	5–20
Parietal cells, of stomach	15–20
Non-parietal cells of stomach	5–7
Bile	4–6
Pancreatic juice	5–15
Succus entericus	4–7
Fresh ileostomy	5–16

3. If urine volume is greater than 600 ml/day, K^+ can be excreted at a rate equal to the ingestion and absorption from a normal diet.
4. In K^+ deficiency, the kidney usually produces an acid urine and retains HCO_3^-, causing a metabolic alkalosis. Occasionally, there is a persistent metabolic acidosis.
5. When glycogen is stored intracellularly, K^+ is stored with it. The reverse is also true; K^+ is released into ECF as glycogen is depleted.
6. K^+ moves out of cells into ECF in any acidosis, and into cells in any alkalosis.

HYPERPOTASSEMIA (HYPERKALEMIA)

Since K^+ can be excreted if urine volume is adequate (see 3 just listed), it follows that severe hyperpotassemia will only occur spontaneously when there is anuria or oliguria with an output of less than 600 ml urine per day.

A mild hyperpotassemia can occur without oliguria in uncontrolled diabetes with acidosis. In this case, there is an overall K^+ deficit developing, but as K^+ moves from the cells into the ECF it is enroute to the kidney where it is excreted. This process can raise the $[K^+]_p$ above normal levels.

PREVENTION

In oliguria or anuria the physician should stop the intake of all food containing K^+. This leaves only purified sugars for oral intake. Some hard candies without soft centers may qualify, but the physician should have the K^+ content checked before allowing the patient to eat them. Sufficient sugars, or intravenous dextrose, should be given to provide the "protein-sparing" action of the carbohydrate intake. If the patient receives no carbohydrates, he will obtain all his caloric needs by burning his own body tissues. As cells are broken down, K^+ is released into the ECF. This process cannot be stopped, but can be reduced to a minimum by administering adequate carbohydrates.

In the adult, 100–150 gm of sugars may be given per day. It is not practical to supply all the patient's caloric requirements with parenteral dextrose or oral sugar intake.

In anuria, it is impossible to prevent the gradual rise of $[K^+]_p$ by following these same procedures, but the rate of rise can be slowed, so that fatal levels are not reached until 7–10 days after the onset of the anuria. Therapy for toxic levels is indicated next.

SIGNS AND SYMPTOMS

The chief symptomatology of hyperpotassemia is related to the cardiovascular system. As $[K^+]_p$ rises, it produces changes in the electrocardiogram. These changes, in the usual order of appearance as the level rises, are:
1. Elevation of the T wave
2. Decrease in size of the R wave
3. Disappearance of the P wave
4. Depression of the S-T segment and widening of the QRS complex
5. Ventricular fibrillation

In addition, gastrointestinal signs and symptoms usually occur. Uremic enteritis often occurs. There may be nausea, intermittent intestinal colic, and/or diarrhea. The diarrhea may be grossly bloody.

TREATMENT

Withhold all K^+, oral and intravenous.

For temporary benefit, to cause K^+ to move from ECF to ICF or to decrease cardiac effects:
1. Intravenous calcium gluconate. This will antagonize the cardiac toxicity of the K^+ without altering the $[K^+]_p$. Dose: up to 30 ml of 10% calcium gluconate added to 250 ml isotonic saline or glucose in water, and administered IV over a 1- to 2-hour period. In a critical patient, the entire 30 ml (3 gm) may be given in 15–30 minutes.
2. Intravenous $NaHCO_3$. The alkalosis produced causes a shift of K^+ from the ECF to the ICF. Dose: 40–160 mEq IV over a 5-minute period. (Do not mix this with the calcium gluconate that is being given, since the bicarbonate will precipitate the calcium.)
3. Intravenous glucose. This is more effective if given with insulin. As the glucose moves intracellularly to be deposited

as glycogen, ECF K^+ moves with it. Dose: 300–500 ml of 20% glucose in H_2O given over a 30–60-minute period. Regular insulin, 1 unit per 2–4 gm of glucose.

If an ECF volume deficit coexists with the hyperpotassemia, then an isotonic salt solution containing no K^+ should be given. This will dilute the ECF $[K^+]$ as the volume deficit is corrected.

To cause loss of K^+ from the body:

1. Ion exchange resins. Sodium polystyrene sulfonate (Kayexalate) is a cation-exchange resin conditioned as the Na^+ salt. In the gastrointestinal tract, the sodium exchanges for potassium, which is then excreted in the stool. The resin may be administered by mouth or by rectum. A laxative is necessary to void fecal impaction. This treatment will not rapidly lower $[K^+]_p$. In anuria, some physicians institute this therapy when $[K^+]_p$ is over 5 mEq/L.

2. Peritoneal dialysis or use of the artificial kidney. The $[K^+]_p$ can be lowered rapidly by these methods. Both of these methods require skilled teams to carry them out. If plasma potassium concentration reaches 7 mEq/L, one of these procedures should be seriously considered, if available.

HYPOPOTASSEMIA (HYPOKALEMIA)

Hypopotassemia is more common than hyperpotassemia.

ETIOLOGY

1. With the loss of any body fluids, K^+ is lost. Because the $[K^+]$ in gastric juice is higher than in other fluids, vomiting causes more loss of K^+ than does a comparable loss of volume of salt water by any other route. Diarrhea, pancreatic fistula, biliary fistula, and sweating all cause K^+ loss. K^+ is not lost at a rapid rate by sweating, and such a loss is usually adequately replaced by food intake.

2. K^+ deficit may result from diabetic hyperglycemia. The loss of K^+ from the body in uncontrolled diabetes was described previously in this chapter. When the hyperglycemia and acidosis are reversed with insulin therapy, glucose is returned to the cells, and stored as glycogen with its accompanying K^+. The $[K^+]_p$ is reduced unless adequate K^+ is administered either orally or parenterally.

3. The modern diuretics used in the treatment of both congestive failure and hypertension are common causes of hypopotassemia. This is particularly true of the thiazide derivatives.
4. There are certain renal diseases associated with tubular dysfunction in which the rate of K^+ loss in the urine is higher than normal. Any patient maintained on parenteral fluids will need K^+ replacement for the normal K^+ loss in the urine.
5. Steroid drugs, particularly the mineralocorticoids, can cause hypopotassemia by increasing the loss in the urine.

SIGNS AND SYMPTOMS OF ACUTE DEFICIT

Hypopotassemia has its effects on the cardiovascular system, CNS, neuromuscular system, the gastrointestinal tract, and the kidney.

CNS.—Disorientation; psychotic behavior.

Skeletal muscle.—Weakness; hypotonic muscles with hypoactive reflexes.

Smooth muscle.—Paralytic ileus with decreased or absent bowel sounds. There is often persistent abdominal distention in spite of nasogastric suction. This is due to decreased propulsive activity.

Cardiovascular.—Changes in the electrocardiogram. These are not sequential with the lowering of $[K^+]_p$. In 80% of the cases the changes are either (1) depression of the S-T segment with a lengthening of the Q-T interval or (2) an inversion of the T wave with lengthening of the Q-T interval. The latter is often associated with the presence of a U wave. Other changes in the ECG which occur less frequently are: (3) upright T wave with prolonged Q-T interval; (4) low amplitude T waves; or (5) prominent U waves with no other abnormality.

Death is by cardiac arrest, with the heart in diastole.

Renal.—Either an associated metabolic alkalosis or metabolic acidosis. In either case, there is an acid urine.

There is impaired ability to concentrate the urine.

Signs and Symptoms of Chronic Deficit

A patient who develops K^+ deficiency slowly, as a complication of diuretic or steroid therapy, may not present all the clinical signs that a patient with an acute deficit manifests. In chronic deficit, weakness is often the chief clinical manifestation. The ECG findings (listed in cardiovascular signs of acute deficit) may or may not be present.

Prevention

Patients with known loss of fluids from the gastrointestinal tract should have adequate K^+ replacement to prevent a deficit from occurring.

Patients taking diuretics known to cause K^+ loss in the urine or patients receiving steroid therapy should have supplemental K^+. This is best given in solution because both pressed and enteric-coated tablets have been shown to cause localized gastrointestinal bleeding. The bleeding is due to local irritation in response to high concentrations of KCl as the tablets dissolve. Details of oral administration are given under the section on treatment.

Treatment

Estimate of Quantity of K^+ To Be Given

The total exchangeable body K^+ of a 70-kg male is about 3,200 mEq. Of this, about 60 mEq is in the ECF. Since deficits of K^+ in the amount of 800–1,000 mEq can occur, it is obvious that the chief deficit is due to K^+ loss from the cells.

Serum K^+ concentration is, therefore, only a rough estimate of the total body K^+ deficit. Since pH changes cause an intracellular-extracellular shift of K^+, the plasma K^+ must be interpreted in light of the pH of the blood. Even this is precarious. For example, an acute respiratory acidosis or alkalosis can cause changes in $[K^+]_p$ without changes in total body K^+.

In cases where the acute disturbance has persisted for 24 hours or longer, it is useful to estimate the total body K^+ deficit from the observed pH and $[K^+]_p$. Table 6–2 gives such estimates for a 70-kg individual. These values would not reflect further losses of K$^+$ from cells that occur in a diabetic who is out of control. There is additional loss of K$^+$ associated with glycogen depletion from the cells.

TABLE 6–2.—K$^+$ DEFICIT AT VARIOUS BLOOD
pH AND [K$^+$]$_p$

[K$^+$]$_p$ (MEQ/L)	BLOOD pH				
	7.0	7.2	7.4	7.6	7.8
2.0	1,550	1,200	960	640	320
3.0	960	710	390	95	0
4.0	640	350	65	0	*
5.0	350	0	*	*	*

*Under these conditions, there is probably some excess total body potassium.

These values are calculated from various values in the literature, based on a 70-kg individual with normal total body potassium of 3,200 mEq.

In diabetes mellitus, the potassium deficit at given conditions is likely to be greater, because of potassium lost as cells are depleted of glycogen.

Route of Administration

Patients acutely ill with K$^+$ deficiency need K$^+$ administered intravenously. Patients with chronic K$^+$ loss from diuretic or steroid therapy may be treated either with oral or intravenous potassium salts.

Intravenous.—The K$^+$ concentration of fluids injected into peripheral veins must not exceed 40 mEq/L, because higher concentrations produce phlebitis. Concentrations of K$^+$ up to 80 mEq/L can be given through a subclavian catheter threaded into the vena cava. The high rate of blood flow in the vena cava prevents high concentrations of K$^+$ from irritating the intima of the vein.

The rate of administration usually should not exceed 20 mEq/hour. When severe K$^+$ deficits are present, rates of 80 mEq/hour may, on rare occasions, be given for a total of 120–160 mEq, after which the rate should be slower.

When total body K^+ depletion of severe degree occurs, even 200 mEq of K^+ administered in the first 24 hours may not result in raising the level of serum K^+ appreciably, but the patient will improve. This improvement is the result of K^+ going intracellularly.

If the patient is on digitalis, intravenous potassium—if used—should be given at slower rates. The digitalis slows the rate of potassium uptake by the cells, and thus makes a transient hyperpotassemia more likely to occur at injection rates of 20 mEq/hour.

Oral.—If oral administration is used, it should be reserved for one of three types of cases: (1) prevention of K^+ deficiency in patients on diuretics or steroids; (2) treatment of moderate degrees of chronic K^+ deficit; or (3) achievement of a final state of normal K^+ balance in acute cases, after IV therapy has returned $[K^+]_p$ to near-normal levels.

A teaspoonful of 25% KCl may be given diluted in water or fruit juice. This contains 13 mEq of K^+. The solution should be given after meals to avoid gastric irritation. Up to 100 mEq/day may be given in severe cases.

MAGNESIUM

Normal plasma magnesium concentration ranges from 1.5 to 2.5 mEq/L. In recent years, the determinations of plasma magnesium have become more readily available in hospitals. It is to be expected that the clinical knowledge of disturbed magnesium metabolism will increase. It is doubtful that the incidence of disturbances will be as great as the incidence of abnormal $[K^+]_p$, but such predictions are not on firm grounds.

PHYSIOLOGIC CONSIDERATIONS

1. Plasma $[Mg^{++}]$ affects the irritability of nervous tissue, and is chiefly manifested by the effects on the CNS. Hypomagnesemia is associated with increased irritability; hypermagnesemia depresses CNS functions.
2. Magnesium is present in most body fluids, so that loss of these produces a loss of magnesium. Particularly important are the succus entericus, bile, and gastric juice.

3. Magnesium is present in high concentrations intracellularly in man and animals. Therefore it is present in meat. It is also present in green vegetables. Normal dietary intake is 25 mEq/day.
4. Magnesium is excreted in the urine even in states of hypomagnesemia.
5. Factors controlling plasma magnesium levels are not well known. The parathyroids play some role, and corticosteroids such as aldosterone have been implicated.

HYPOMAGNESEMIA

Etiology

1. Chronic alcoholism. This is an empirical fact, and the mechanism of production is not well established. Increased loss in the urine due to the alcohol is known to occur.
2. Prolonged parenteral fluid therapy without Mg^{++} in fluids. In this situation the Mg^{++} loss is due to renal excretion.
3. Renal disease. Hypomagnesemia occurs especially in chronic renal diseases such as glomerulonephritis and pyelonephritis before severe azotemia occurs. The mechanism is excessive loss in the urine. In the late stages of these diseases, the reverse is true; magnesium is not excreted and [Mg^{++}]$_p$ increases.
4. Acute renal tubular disease during the diuretic phase. Again, the mechanism is loss of Mg^{++} in the urine.
5. Chronic diarrhea. There is a loss of Mg^{++} in the feces, and there may also be malabsorption of Mg^{++} from the diet.
6. Chronic biliary fistulas, and nasogastric suction with inadequate replacement.

Signs and Symptoms

Decrease in [Mg^{++}]$_p$ causes an increased irritability of nervous tissue. This irritability most often mimics a convulsive disorder. When death is caused by hypomagnesemia, it often occurs during a convulsion. Tetanic manifestations similar to those occurring with hypocalcemia have been described. If these occur in a known case of hypomagnesemia, one should make sure that a hypocalcemia does not coexist.

LABORATORY FINDINGS

A magnesium level less than 1.5 mEq/L should be treated if the clinical history is consistent with hypomagnesemia. A serum calcium should also be obtained.

PREVENTION

A patient losing fluids from the intestinal or biliary tract over a long period of time should have 2–3 mEq/L of Mg^{++} included in the salt solutions used for replacement of saltwater loss.

TREATMENT

Specific treatment of hypomagnesemia requires Mg^{++} replacement. Three routes of treatment are available.

1. Oral. Unless there is malabsorption, this method should be tried initially in moderate cases. Dietary Mg^{++} can be supplemented by administering 2 gm (33 mEq) of $MgSO_4$ up to 3 times a day without producing diarrhea.
2. Intramuscular. Two grams of $MgSO_4$ in solution (4 ml of 50% solution) can be given as often as 4 times daily for 3–5 days.
3. Intravenous. One liter of 160 mEq/L $MgSO_4$ in 5% dextrose in water can be given intravenously over a period of 2–4 hours. This is 1% $MgSO_4$ and is made by adding 20 ml of 50% $MgSO_4$ to a liter of 5% dextrose in water. This method should be used only in severe cases where the diagnosis is certain.

HYPERMAGNESEMIA

ETIOLOGY

1. Chronic renal disease with severe azotemia. The mechanism is failure of the kidney to excrete Mg^{++}.
2. Associated with untreated diabetic acidosis. The mechanism is release of intracellular Mg^{++} into the ECF.
3. Occasional cases due to oral administration of Mg^{++} salts, or the use of $MgSO_4$ enemas. This is especially likely to occur in patients with impaired renal function.
4. Hyperparathyroidism.

SIGNS AND SYMPTOMS

The chief clinical feature is depression of CNS function. As the plasma level rises there is first lethargy. Coma eventually occurs and death is most often a result of respiratory failure. Correlation of these events with plasma Mg^{++} levels is not well documented. Death most likely occurs at plasma levels above 6 mEq/L.

Excess Mg^{++} does affect the heart. The ECG may show prolonged P-R intervals, and a prolonged ventricular complex.

PROPHYLAXIS

The intake of medications containing Mg^{++} should be avoided in patients with severe azotemia. Chiefly, these would be MgSO$_4$ and antacids containing Mg^{++}.

TREATMENT

The treatment of hypermagnesemia is not clear cut. The following principles may be helpful:

1. If there is an associated milliosmolar concentration and/or ECF volume deficit, this should be corrected using fluids which do not contain Mg^{++} and which thereby dilute the Mg^{++} in the ECF.
2. If the cause of the hypermagnesemia is untreated diabetic acidosis, the specific treatment of the acidosis will probably be adequate.
3. In end-stage renal disease, the artificial kidney or peritoneal dialysis is the only satisfactory long-term therapy.
4. If no cause of hypermagnesemia is apparent, hyperparathyroid disease should be ruled out.
5. The depressant effects of hypermagnesemia can be antagonized by intravenous administration of calcium salts. The mechanism of this action is not apparent.

BIBLIOGRAPHY

ON POTASSIUM

Burnell, J. M., *et al.*: The effect in humans of extracellular pH change on the relationship between serum potassium concentration and intracellular potassium, J. Clin. Invest. 35:935, 1956.

Chamberlain, M. J.: Emergency treatment of hyperkalaemia, Lancet 1:464, 1964.

Clementsen, H. J.: Potassium therapy; a break with tradition, Lancet 2:175, 1962.

Hopper, J., O'Connell, B. P., and Fluss, H. R.: Serum potassium patterns in anuria and oliguria, Ann. Intern. Med. 38:935, 1953.

Knowles, H. C., Jr., and Kaplan, S. A.: Treatment of hyperkalemia in acute renal failure using exchange resins, Arch. Intern. Med. 92:189, 1953.

Scherr, L., et al.: Management of hyperkalemia with a cation-exchange resin, N. Engl. J. Med. 264:115, 1961.

Surawicz, B., et al.: Clinical manifestations of hypopotassemia, Am. J. Med. Sci. 233:603, 1957.

Weaver, W. F., and Burchell, H. B.: Serum potassium and the electrocardiogram in hypokalemia, Circulation 21:505, 1960.

ON MAGNESIUM

Aikawa, J. K.: *The Role of Magnesium in Biologic Processes* (Springfield, Ill.: Charles C Thomas, 1963).

Flink, E. B.: Magnesium deficiency in man, J.A.M.A. 160:1406, 1956.

Randall, R. E., Jr., et al.: Hypermagnesemia in renal failure, etiology and toxic manifestations, Ann. Intern. Med. 61:73, 1964.

Wacker, W. E. C., and Parisi, A. F.: Magnesium metabolism, N. Engl. J. Med. 278:658, 712 and 772, 1968.

Zimmet, P., Breidahl, H. D., and Nayler, W. G.: Plasma ionized calcium in hypomagnesaemia, Br. Med. J. 1:622, 1968

7 / Diagnosis and Therapy of Compound Disturbances of Fluid and Electrolyte Balance

ASSUMING that the reader has developed a familiarity with the signs and symptoms of relatively simple disturbances of concentration, volume, and composition, the present chapter offers a discussion of compound and mixed disturbances and their clinical and therapeutic relationships. The aim is not to encompass all major disturbances, but to demonstrate the principles involved in diagnosis and treatment.

` The following principles of therapy, while not without exception, have proven to be safe and direct in the treatment of multiple disturbances:

1. When multiple deficits occur, the correction of osmolar concentration should take precedence.
2. The rate of restoration of ECF volume depletion must be correlated with the clinical history. A patient with an acute saltwater loss, such as occurs in burns, peritonitis, or shock, needs rapid volume replacement. A patient with a deficit developing gradually might be overloaded by rapid infusion of salt water.
3. The clinical state takes precedence over the laboratory findings in diagnosis and treatment.
4. Changes in fluid and electrolyte balance are usually the result of other derangements and—while therapy to restore normal volume, concentration, and composition is critical—it also follows that treatment of the primary diseases must take place concomitantly.

VOMITING

In diagnosing the water balance disturbance in a patient who is vomiting, one must consider the possible different losses by this route.

The pyloric glands produce gastric secretions high in K^+ and with significant Na^+ content. The $[K^+]$ is about 15 mEq/L.

The secretion from the parietal cells is isotonic, but contains chiefly hydrocholoric acid. The $[K^+]$ is 5–8 mEq/L. In the formation of hydrochloric acid, sodium bicarbonate is returned to the ECF. If there is continued vomiting of the acid, the ECF will become more alkaline.

In some patients who have been vomiting for a long period of time, the pyloric sphincter relaxes, and large quantities of alkaline duodenal contents are lost. These patients will usually have bile in the vomitus.

Consider a patient who vomits repeatedly over a period of several days and takes no food or fluids during this time. The vomitus is very acid when tested with pH paper, indicating that the individual is producing HCl, and that the loss of duodenal secretion is unlikely.

One would then predict a decrease in the ECF volume due to the saltwater loss. In addition, the concentration of body fluids would increase because of insensible water loss with no replacement. There would be compositional changes. The vomiting would produce a metabolic alkalosis, a potassium loss, and some loss of magnesium. Unless the vomiting persists for a long time, symptoms of magnesium loss will not become apparent.

CLINICAL PICTURE OF ECF VOLUME DEFICIT WITH WATER DEFICIT, METABOLIC ALKALOSIS, AND POTASSIUM DEFICIT

History
    A. Vomiting with no food or fluid intake
    B. Weakness due to both the ECF volume loss and K^+ loss
    C. Dizziness except when recumbent
    D. Syncope
Physical Examination
    A. Blood pressure hypotensive. (The severity depends upon the volume of salt deficit.)
    B. Temperature increased. (Fever may be present; however, if the water deficit is mild and saltwater deficit severe hypothermia might exist.)
    C. Skin turgor reduced
    D. CNS signs the same as for an ECF volume deficit

Laboratory Findings
  A. Blood and plasma
     1. The pH would be on the alkaline side of normal, primarily because of vomiting. The starvation would tend to produce an acidosis, but this would be more than offset by the vomiting.
     2. $[HCO_3^-]_p$ would be elevated because of both the metabolic alkalosis and the concentrating effect of the simple water loss.
     3. $[Na^+]_p$ and osmolality by freezing-point depression would be elevated only because of the water loss. The saltwater loss does not change the $[Na^+]_p$.
     4. $[K^+]_p$ would be reduced. The vomiting would markedly reduce the K^+ content of the body, and the alkalosis would move K^+ into cells.
  B. Urine
     1. Volume would be reduced. Two factors operate to cause oliguria. The hyperosmolality causes ADH release with a consequent oliguria, and the ECF volume deficit reduces the glomerular filtration rate. A severe saltwater deficit can produce anuria.
     2. Specific gravity would be increased. If the patient had normal renal function before the onset of vomiting, the sp. gr. would be greater than 1.025.
     3. Initially the urine pH would be alkaline as the kidney excretes bicarbonate in an attempt to correct the alkalosis. As the condition progresses, the urine becomes acid (the potassium deficiency causes an inappropriate acidification of the urine).

TREATMENT

1. Five per cent glucose in water for the water deficit.
2. An isotonic salt solution for the saltwater deficit. Lactate or bicarbonate are contraindicated. Sodium chloride (0.9%) will dilute the high $[HCO_3^-]_p$. If the alkalosis is severe, 1/6 M NH_4Cl can be given intravenously.
3. One must weigh the severity of the hypopotassemia against the severity of the oliguria to determine when large

amounts of potassium salts should be added to the therapy.

As stated previously, treatment of the water deficit takes precedence over the treatment of the ECF deficit. Often 2.5% glucose in half-isotonic (0.45%) saline can be given. Rates of glucose administration exceeding 3 gm per hour are likely to produce glycosuria.

As a rough guide to the volume of water (as opposed to salt water) needed, one can use the following calculation:

$$\frac{\% \text{ elevation of } [Na^+] \text{ above normal}}{100} \times$$
weight in kg $\times$ 0.60 water = liters of water deficit

For example, if the $[Na^+]_p$ is 156 mEq/L in a 70-kg individual, the elevation of $[Na^+]_p$ is then 10%.

$$\frac{10}{100} \times 70 \text{ kg} \times 0.60 = 4.2L, \text{ the approximate water deficit}$$

In treating the patient, this volume plus the calculated insensible loss during the treatment period should be considered. The estimates are never firm enough to take the place of frequent observations of the patient, and of appropriate laboratory studies during the treatment.

There is no good estimate of the degree of saltwater depletion. It is important to remember that in a 70-kg individual, clinical signs do not appear until a deficit of about 3 liters is present. After some experience in treating such cases, the clinician will develop a judgment as to the amount of salt water that will be needed.

Synonyms: ECF volume deficit with increased osmolar concentration; ECF volume deficit with intracellular fluid volume deficit; or ECF volume deficit with simple water deficit. (These synonyms do not include the compositional disturbances of the case just discussed.)

CLINICAL PICTURE OF ECF VOLUME DEFICIT WITH COMPENSATED RESPIRATORY ACIDOSIS

This case is presented to emphasize that a patient may not be in normal water and electrolyte balance before the onset of an illness which brings him to the physician.

This is the clinical picture in a patient with chronic lung disease, such as emphysema, who develops a severe diarrhea.

History
- A. Diarrhea
- B. Dyspnea on exertion, but no orthopnea (This is due to the respiratory disease.)
- C. Weakness due to the ECF volume depletion
- D. Dizziness
- E. Syncope

Physical Examination
- A. Blood pressure hypotensive (The severity depends upon the volume of saltwater deficit.)
- B. Body temperature reduced if environmental temperature below 65–70 F
- C. Skin turgor reduced
- D. CNS signs same as for ECF deficit
- E. Clinical and roentgenologic signs of chronic pulmonary disease

Laboratory Findings
- A. Blood and plasma
  1. pH would be on the acid-side of normal, both because of diarrhea and because of the respiratory disease.
  2. $[HCO_3^-]_p$ would be elevated because of the compensation for the respiratory acidosis.
  3. $[Na^+]_p$ would be normal. Such a case might actually be complicated by either a water deficit or a water excess, with the appropriate disturbance in $[Na^+]_p$.
  4. $[K^+]_p$ would be normal, or slightly decreased, because of diarrhea.
- B. Urine
  1. Volume would be normal or slightly reduced.
  2. pH would probably be below 5.5. The kidney initially had compensated for the respiratory acidosis. The diarrhea tends to reduce the already elevated $[HCO_3^-]_p$, thus decreasing compensation. Whether the term metabolic acidosis would apply in this case is only a semantic problem. In any event, the kidney must once again retain bicarbonate, and excrete an acid urine to regain maximum compensation.

TREATMENT

It is important to recognize the compensated respiratory acidosis. Salt water must be administered without significantly reducing the $[HCO_3^-]_p$. Isotonic saline is contraindicated. Lactated Ringer's solution should be given in an amount sufficient to correct the signs of the ECF volume depletion.

CHRONIC WATER DEFICIT

Of special interest is the syndrome produced by chronic water deficit. This is seen in a limited number of patients, such as disturbed or aged persons in chronic-care facilities.

These patients may drink water, but not have adequate intake. They then produce some urine, but are in a state of chronic, mild hyperosmolality. Under these conditions, the urine is concentrated and contains a large amount of sodium salts. The gradual depletion of the sodium content of the body results in ECF volume reduction. This results in CNS depression, and the patient drinks even less water.

The result is a combined water deficit and a saltwater deficit. However, the route of the loss of salt water is occult. It is lost through an otherwise normal kidney.

8 / Cases for Diagnosis and Treatment

THE FOLLOWING are theoretical cases for the reader to diagnose, and then to outline the principles of treatment. Such cases have been found useful in teaching Moyer's method of diagnosing a patient with disturbed water and electrolyte balance.

The first case is analyzed in detail, and Table 8–1 suggests a manner in which the beginner might sort out the history, signs, symptoms, and laboratory findings in a useful manner.

CASE 1

A 33-year-old white male, weight 75 kg.—It is July with an ambient daytime temperature of 95–100 F (35–38 C). The patient gives a history of chronic duodenal peptic ulcer. He has been vomiting for 5 days, and has taken no food. He has drunk some water but vomits 20–30 minutes after drinking. He complains of extreme weakness.

Vital signs.—T, 101 F (38.3 C); P, 115/minute; R, 14/minute; BP, 88/45 recumbent.

Relevant physical findings.—Patient is lethargic. Loss of skin turgor. During the examination he shows mild carpopedal spasm.

Laboratory findings.—Blood: pH, 7.52; P_{CO_2}, 60 mm Hg; Hb, 14 gm/100 ml.
Plasma: (in mEq/L) $[Na^+]$, 160; $[K^+]$, 3.2; $[Mg^{++}]$, 1.6; $[HCO_3^-]$, 50.0; delta base, plus 21.0; $[Cl^-]$, 90. Osmolality, 310 mOsm/kg water.
Urine: sample unobtainable.
ECG: shows low voltage.

Diagnosis

1. Water deficit with hyperosmolality
2. Saltwater deficit with decreased ECF volume

TABLE 8–1.—ORGANIZATION OF DATA FROM CASE 1

	WATER GAIN OR LOSS (CONCENTRATION)	SALTWATER GAIN, OR LOSS (VOLUME)	ACID-BASE	K^+	Mg^{++}
History	Hot environment* Drinks water and vomits† Presumably no food intake	Vomiting, plus vomiting after drinking†	Peptic ulcer plus vomiting†	Hot environment* Vomiting†	Vomiting*
Signs and symptoms	T, 101 F	T, 101F Loss of skin turgor Hypotension	Carpopedal spasm	Oliguria Weakness	
Laboratory	Na^+, 160 mEq/L, Osmolality, 310 mOsm/kg water, Oliguria	Oliguria	Blood pH, 7.52 HCO_3^-, 50.0 mEq/L Delta base, plus 21.0 mEq/L Anion gap: $Na^+ + K^+$ 163.2 $HCO_3^- + Cl^-$ 150.0 13.2	K^+, 3.2 mEq/L pH, 7.48 ECG, low voltage	Mg^{++}, 1.6 mEq/L

*Hot environment suggests an increase in the insensible loss plus sweating. This will cause a loss of water and K^+. In July, one would expect the patient to be acclimatized to the heat, and so Na^+ loss would be low.

†The vomiting represents a loss of salt water. With a history of peptic ulcer, one would assume the patient produced HCl, and vomiting would cause an alkalosis. The drinking of water and then vomiting cause a further saltwater loss, but represent a factor that is diluting the body fluids.

3. Metabolic alkalosis, probably compensated
4. Hypopotassemia
5. Normal magnesium

Comment

1. The history suggests a water deficit, but one cannot predict the degree of hyperosmolality the patient would have. He has not gained any water from eating food, and probably has gained very little from the drinking. The fever and oliguria are compatible with a water deficit. The elevated plasma Na^+ and osmolality establish the diagnosis.
2. The history indicates a saltwater loss. There is no apparent replacement. The hypotension and decreased skin turgor further strengthen the diagnosis. The laboratory tests recorded are of no help. Remember that there are no diagnostic laboratory tests which firmly establish a decrease in ECF volume. A low urine $[Na^+]$ or $[Cl^-]$ would be expected if a urine sample could be obtained.
3. As stated, the vomiting in a patient with known peptic ulcer is strong evidence that there is HCl loss in the vomitus. This will produce a metabolic alkalosis. The blood pH, plasma $[HCO_3^-]$, and delta base establish this diagnosis. The elevated Pco_2 is evidence for a compensation of the alkalosis. The mechanism producing the carpopedal spasm is a depression of the ionized calcium by the alkalosis.
4. The vomiting represents a large loss of K^+. The loss in sweat is small in comparison. The low plasma $[K^+]$ must be interpreted in light of the acid-base disturbance. Referring to Table 6–2, one would estimate the deficit to be a little less than 300 mEq. Oliguria is listed under K^+ because it is a factor to consider in treatment.
5. There are no symptoms to suggest a disturbance in Mg^{++}, and the plasma concentration is normal. There is some Mg^{++} in vomitus, but the condition has not existed for a sufficient length of time to cause a large loss.

Treatment

1. The patient should receive calcium gluconate intravenously because of his carpopedal spasm.

2. Both water and salt water should be given. This can be done by administering half-strength 5% glucose in saline intravenously to replace sodium volume and reduce osmolar concentration. Volume alone, once osmolar concentration has been corrected, can be treated with 0.9% sodium chloride or Ringer's solution, which would also correct the metabolic alkalosis. Lactated Ringer's solution should not be given, because it is desirable to dilute the high bicarbonate.

3. The K^+ deficiency is not severe or life threatening. By using Ringer's solution, plasma K^+ will not be significantly diluted, and some K^+ will come out of cells as the alkalosis is corrected. Eventually, higher concentrations of KCl will be needed in the IV solutions to correct the deficit. It is a matter of judgment to decide whether this should be initiated before the anuria is reversed. Certainly, when urine flow becomes greater than 600 ml/24 hours, then KCl should be added in concentrations of 40 mEq/L to one of the solutions. Plasma $[K^+]$ should be monitored throughout treatment.

4. The metabolic alkalosis is not severe. The effects of dilution plus the improved renal function would be expected to correct the situation.

CASE 2

A 63-year-old black male, weight 87 kg.—This patient had a severe myocardial infarction 2 years ago, and is now maintained on digitalis and a thiazide diuretic. He has had mild diarrhea for 3 days, during which time he continued to take water by mouth, but no food.

Vital signs.—T, 97.8 F (36.6 C); P, 88/minute; R, 13/minute; BP, 115/65 recumbent, 110/50 sitting.

Relevant physical findings.—Patient is sleepy. Decreased skin turgor; hypoactive knee reflexes; hypotonic muscles.

Laboratory findings.—Blood: pH, 7.38; Pco_2, 36 mm Hg; Hb, 13.6 gm/100 ml.
Plasma: (in mEq/L) $[Na^+]$, 140; $[K^+]$, 2.8; $[Mg^{++}]$, 1.7; $[HCO_3^-]$, 21.0; delta base, minus 3; $[Cl^-]$, 109. Osmolality, 288 mOsm/kg water.

Urine: voided 200 ml at time of examination; sp. gr., 1.016; pH, 5.0.

Diagnosis and analysis on pages 99–100.

CASE 3

An oriental male estimated to be 60–65 years old, weight about 60 kg.—The patient was brought in by ambulance in response to a neighbor's call. The neighbors had not seen him for about 4 days. Before that, he was active, working in his yard every day. It is October and the weather has been mild.

Vital signs.—T, 95.5 F (35.3 C); P, thready, 125/minute; R, 11/minute; BP, 86/50 recumbent.

Relevant physical findings.—The patient is unconscious and responds to painful stimuli by withdrawing limbs. His mouth is dry. There is marked loss of skin turgor. Abdomen is rigid; no bowel sounds are heard.

Laboratory findings.—Blood: pH, 7.43; Pco_2, 43 mm Hg; Hb, 12.0 gm/100 ml; urea N, 50 mg/100 ml.
Plasma: (in mEq/L) [Na^+], 160; [K^+], 5.7; [Mg^{++}], 2.3; [HCO_3^-], 28.5; delta base, plus 4; [Cl^-], 116. Osmolality, 316 mOsm/kg water.
Urine: 20 ml obtained by catheter: sp. gr., 1.031.

Diagnosis and analysis on pages 100–101.

CASE 4

A 68-year-old white male, estimated weight 80 kg.—This patient is in a semicomatose condition, brought into the hospital by his son. He has had symptoms of urethral obstruction for at least 2 years. Food intake was poor during the last 7 weeks. Because of fear of going to a physician he has not sought medical help previous to this.

Vital signs.—T, 99.2 F (37.3 C); P, 114/minute; R, 14/minute; BP, 105/60, recumbent.

Relevant physical findings.—The patient is semicomatose. His mouth is dry. Decreased skin turgor.

Laboratory findings. — Blood: pH, 7.35; P_{CO_2}, 32.0 mm Hg; Hb, 10 gm/100 ml; urea N, 337 mg/100 ml.

Plasma: (in mEq/L) [Na$^+$], 114; [K$^+$], 8.8; [Mg^{++}], 2.2; [HCO$_3^-$], 17.6; delta base, minus 7; [Cl$^-$], 86; [Ca^{++}] 3.6. Osmolality, 342 mOsm/kg water.

Urine: no sample obtained.

ECG: absence of P waves, and abnormal T waves with depression of the S-T segment and widening of the QRS complexes.

Diagnosis and analysis on pages 101–103.

CASE 5

A 32-year-old Latin-American female, weight 60 kg. — This lady was recently diagnosed as having diabetes insipidus, and treatment with antidiuretic hormone was begun. Fluid intake was not restricted. About 24 hours after the onset of therapy, the patient convulsed. She vomited once, and has had a couple of loose stools. The patient complains of a severe headache.

Vital signs. — T, 98.4 F (36.9 C); P, 60/minute; R, 13/minute; BP, 150/95.

Relevant physical findings. — Excessive lacrimation; fingerprint edema over sternum; hyperactive tendon reflexes.

Laboratory findings. — Blood: pH, 7.38; P_{CO_2}, 38 mm Hg; Hb, 13.8 gm/100 ml.

Plasma: (in mEq/L) [Na$^+$], 119; [K$^+$], 3.6; [Mg^{++}], 1.7; [HCO$_3^-$], 22.5; delta base, minus 2.0; [Cl$^-$], 86. Osmolality, 234 mOsm/kg water.

Urine: volume, 100 ml estimated to have been produced in 2 hours; sp. gr., 1.025; pH, 6.5.

Diagnosis and analysis on pages 103–104.

CASE 6

A 27-year-old black female, weight 57 kg. — This patient has been admitted for diagnostic procedures because of unexplained abdominal discomfort after eating. She gives no history of excessive gain or loss of fluids.

Vital signs.—T, 98.6 F (37.0 C); P, 76/minute; R, 12/minute; BP, 124/84 sitting.

Relevant physical findings.—There are no specific signs of water and electrolyte disturbances.

Laboratory findings.—Blood: pH, 7.40; PCO_2, 39 mm Hg; Hb, 14.2 gm/100 ml.
Plasma: (in mEq/L) [Na+], 123; [K+], 3.3; [Mg++], 1.8; [HCO_3^-], 24.0; delta base, minus 1, [Cl−], 87. Osmolality, 280 mOsm/kg water. The laboratory reports that the plasma is not clear, but milky.
Urine: sp. gr., 1.018; pH, 6.5.

Diagnosis and analysis on pages 104–105.

CASE 7

A 58-year-old white male, weight 75 kg.—This man has a diagnosis of advanced emphysema. He developed diarrhea, with loose watery stools. He took nothing by mouth for 2 days.

Vital signs.—T, 97.0 F (36.1 C); P, 94/minute; R, 18/minute; BP, 120/78 recumbent, 90/62 sitting.

Relevant physical findings.—The patient is sleepy, but when aroused he knows his name. However he quickly falls off to sleep again. Barrel-shaped chest. Decrease in skin turgor.

Laboratory findings.—Blood: pH, 7.28; PCO_2, 83 mm Hg; Hb, 16.0 gm/100 ml.
Plasma: (in mEq/L) [Na+], 150; [K+], 4.0; [Mg++], 1.9; [HCO_3^-], 38.5; delta base, plus 7; [Cl−], 104. Osmolality, 310 mOsm/kg water.
Urine: estimated urine flow of 50 ml in 2 hours; sp. gr., 1.034; pH, 4.7.

Diagnosis and analysis on pages 105–106.

CASE 8

A 42-year-old white female, weight 66 kg.—This is a known diabetic admitted in a semicomatose state.

Vital signs.—T, 97.0 F (36.1 C); P, 115/minute; R, 14/minute; BP, 90/50 recumbent.

Relevant physical findings.—Decreased skin turgor; soft eyeballs.

Laboratory findings.—Blood: pH, 7.39; P_{CO_2}, 43 mm Hg; Hb, 13.8 gm/100 ml; glucose, 1,490 mg/100 ml.
Plasma: (in mEq/L) [Na^+], 140; [K^+], 5.3; [Mg^{++}], 1.8; [HCO_3^-], 26; delta base, plus 1; [Cl^-], 102. Osmolality, 363 mOsm/kg water.
Urine: marked diuresis, with estimated 200 ml in the last hour. Sugar, 4+; sp. gr., 1.054; pH, 6.50. Tests for acetone and ketone bodies are negative.

Diagnosis and analysis on pages 107–108

CASE 9

A 68-year-old white female, weight 63 kg.—This patient is seen in consultation. She has had continuous nasogastric suction for 14 days following abdominal surgery. She has had adequate Na^+, K^+, and water replacement.

Vital signs.—T, 101.2 F (37.3 C); P, 90/minute; R, 14/minute; BP, 125/85.

Relevant physical findings.—The patient is disoriented as to time and place. Athetoid and choreiform movements, with muscle twitchings. Normal skin turgor.

Laboratory findings.—Blood: pH, 7.39; P_{CO_2}, 39 mm Hg; Hb, 12.0 gm/100 ml.
Plasma: (in mEq/L) [Na^+], 145; [K^+], 4.2; [Mg^{++}], 0.67; [Ca^{++}], 4.5; [HCO_3^-], 23.5; delta base, plus 1; [Cl^-], 104. Osmolality, 287 mOsm/kg water.
Urine: volume, 1,250 ml in last 24 hours; sp. gr., 1.016.

Diagnosis and analysis on page 108.

CASE 10

A 17-year-old white female, weight 58 kg.—The patient complains of weakness, tiredness, and dyspnea on exertion. She has had recurrent black, tarry stools for about a month.

Vital signs.—T, 98.4 F (36.9 C); P, 114/minute; R, 18/minute; BP, 110/70.

Relevant physical findings.—Pale mucous membranes. Normal skin turgor.

Laboratory findings.—Blood: pH, 7.47; Pco_2, 27.5 mm Hg; Hb, 4.5 gm/100 ml.

Plasma: (in mEq/L) $[Na^+]$, 141; $[K^+]$, 3.5; $[Mg^{++}]$, 1.6; $[HCO_3^-]$, 20; delta base, minus 3.5; $[Cl^-]$, 111. Osmolality, 278 mOsm/kg water.

Urine: voided 250 ml; sp. gr., 1.018; pH, 7.50.

Diagnosis and analysis on page 109.

DIAGNOSIS AND TREATMENT OF CASES 2–10

CASE 2

Diagnosis

1. Normal concentration
2. Saltwater deficit with decreased ECF volume
3. Very mild metabolic acidosis, compensated
4. Hypopotassemia, severe
5. Normal magnesium

Comment

The lethargy, decreased skin turgor, hypothermia, and hypotension are signs of a decreased ECF volume. The route of loss of salt water is obviously diarrhea.

The mild acidosis is most probably due to HCO_3^- in the stools. In an adult, starvation is not likely to have produced much acidosis in 2 days. If this diagnosis were omitted, it would not be a serious error.

The hypopotassemia is severe and is primarily due to the administration of diuretics. The diarrhea would cause additional loss of K^+. One would estimate the deficit to be in the range of 400–500 mEq.

Treatment

1. The patient needs an isotonic salt solution, preferably lactated Ringer's solution. This would prevent further

lowering of both HCO_3^- and K^+ concentrations. Because of the cardiac status, the rate of administration should be slow.

2. Water by mouth may be given ad lib. If the patient cannot drink water, then sufficient 5% glucose in water should be given IV to maintain insensible loss.

3. Supplemental potassium salts must be given. Because the patient is digitalized, K^+ must be administered slowly, at a rate less than 20 mEq/hour. The K^+ in the Ringer's lactate solution could be increased to 40 mEq/L and given over a 3–4-hour period. The deficit should be corrected slowly over at least 5–6 days. After the saltwater deficit has been corrected, it would be best to give a KCl solution by mouth.

CASE 3

Diagnosis

1. Severe water deficit with hyperosmolality
2. Saltwater deficit (probably a distributional shift due to peritonitis)
3. Acid-base state normal when corrected for the effects of the water deficit on $[HCO_3^-]$
4. Hyperpotassemia, partly due to the hyperosmolality
5. Normal magnesium

Comment

It is probable that this patient did not eat a great deal or partake of any fluids for several days prior to admission to the hospital. The plasma $[Na^+]$ and osmolality both indicate an increased milliosmolar concentration, and the magnitude is about 13%. This represents a deficit of about 5.5 liters of water (60 kg × 0.70 normal fraction of water × 0.13 fractional loss).

The comatose state observed could be due to many causes. With the hypotension and decreased skin turgor, a saltwater deficit is likely. With no evidence of an external loss of salt water, an internal loss would be suspected. The rigid abdomen and absence of bowel sounds suggest a peritonitis. Although neither diagnosis is proved, the evidence of a saltwater deficit is sufficient to initiate saltwater replacement.

In interpreting both $[HCO_3^-]$ and $[K^+]$ in the presence of a severe water deficit, one must remember that these will be diluted as the deficit is corrected. Reducing these values by about 13% places them in normal range.

Treatment

The osmolar concentration can be corrected by administration of 5% glucose in water. The volume to be given depends upon the response of the patient, but it could be estimated to be 2–4 liters during the first 2 hours of therapy. After the concentration is corrected, volume depletion can be made up with lactated Ringer's solution. A sufficient volume should be given to correct the clinical signs present.

CASE 4

Diagnosis

1. Water deficit with hyperosmolality
2. Saltwater deficit
3. Metabolic acidosis
4. Hyperpotassemia
5. Normal magnesium
6. Uremia

Comment

1. The history is difficult to evaluate, but it must be presumed that the patient went into a semicomatose state and did not eat or drink. This would produce a water deficit. The osmolality establishes the diagnosis. Even without this, diagnosis could be made by calculating the osmolality increase due to the elevated urea:

$$\frac{(337 - 15) \times 10}{28} = 115 \text{ mOsm/L due to the elevation in urea.}$$

$115 \div 2 = 57.5$, call it 58 mEq of Na salts
to produce the same number of mOsm/L.

The 58 is then added to 114 mEq/L of Na, and compared with the normal value of 142 mEq/L. The high total of 172 indicates a water deficit.

2. The saltwater deficit has occurred because of the vomiting, with possibly some loss from the kidney. The decrease in skin turgor, and the low blood pressure support this diagnosis. The temperature is elevated, but since there is the possibility of a low-grade urinary tract infection, one would not expect the hypothermia that often accompanies a saltwater deficit.

3. There are several factors in the patient's history which could contribute to a disturbed acid-base state. A metabolic acidosis is usually associated with uremia. Starvation could produce a metabolic acidosis. The history is not conclusive.

The laboratory findings show that the patient is slightly acidotic, as indicated by the blood pH. The P_{CO_2} indicates that it is a compensated metabolic acidosis. The $[HCO_3^-]$ is affected by two factors other than acid-base balance. Just as $[Na^+]$ is reduced by the osmotic effect of the urea, the $[HCO_3^-]$ and $[Cl^-]$ would be likewise reduced. The water deficit would be a factor increasing the concentration of all ions. Calculations for these effects should be made before interpreting the severity of the acid-base state. The delta-base figure is not a reliable index of the degree of the disturbance in this case.

Since $[Na^+]$ has also been affected by these two factors, how a normal $[HCO_3^-]$ would be affected can be calculated by using a simple proportion:

$$\frac{\text{normal } [Na^+]}{\text{observed } [Na^+]} = \frac{\text{normal } [HCO_3^-]}{X}$$

$$\frac{142}{114} = \frac{27.0}{21.6}$$

where X is the expected value for $[HCO_3^-]$ if there were no acid-base disturbance. Since the observed $[HCO_3^-]$ is 17.6 mEq/L, it is lower than would be predicted if there were normal acid-base balance.

4. The hyperpotassemia is secondary to the disturbed renal function, and the ECG is consistent with this diagnosis.

Treatment

It is assumed that the patient is to be treated until dialysis, either by the artificial kidney or by peritoneal lavage, can be instituted.

1. Calcium gluconate IV should be given as soon as possible.
2. This patient needs glucose with insulin. Give 5% glucose in water IV rapidly with insulin.
3. Five percent glucose in water should be given, and the amount to give is best followed by repeated determinations of plasma osmolality.
4. Give 40–160 mEq of $NaHCO_3$ as an isotonic solution.
5. The patient needs salt water, but no K^+, so both Ringer's solution and lactated Ringer's solution are contraindicated. A solution of 0.9% NaCl with 27 mEq/L sodium lactate added should be given. This will replace the saltwater deficit without adding to the dilution.
6. If dialysis cannot be started promptly, give an ion exchange resin by mouth.

CASE 5

Diagnosis

1. Simple water excess with milliosmolar dilution
2. Normal ECF volume
3. Acid-base balance that will be normal when dilution is corrected
4. Normal potassium
5. Normal magnesium

Comment

The $[Na^+]$ and osmolality indicate a water excess. The urine specific gravity is high because the administered antidiuretic hormone has prevented the normal concentrating-diluting mechanisms from responding to this water excess. The convulsion, fingerprint edema, and elevated blood pressure are all symptoms compatible with the water excess.

This is not an unusual occurrence in instituting treatment of diabetes insipidus. In these individuals, the drinking of large quantities of water is such a habit that they continue the high intake even though it is inappropriate for the body's needs.

The vomiting and loose stools are symptoms of a water excess. These fluids will contain salt. Since there are no signs present that indicate a saltwater deficit, the quantity lost by these routes must not have been great.

The $[HCO_3^-]$, $[K^+]$, and $[Mg^{++}]$ must be calculated to determine the values they will have when the dilution is corrected to normal. They would become 26 mEq/L, 4.3 mEq/L, and 2.0 mEq/L, respectively. Therefore the composition of the ECF is normal.

Treatment

1. Withhold intake of fluids by mouth, and give no 5% glucose in water parenterally.
2. Stop further administration of antidiuretic hormone.
3. Administer 100 ml 5% NaCl IV over a 1-hour period. If there are further convulsive episodes, the rate could be increased. After completion, observe for at least 1/2 hour, and repeat if necessary.
4. When diuresis occurs due to the withholding of ADH, repeat the laboratory determination of osmolality, or $[Na^+]$. When these rise to normal values, resume treatment with ADH, but limit fluid intake to 1.5 L/day if the patient can eat.

CASE 6

Diagnosis

The concentration, volume, and composition of ECF are all in normal range.

Comment

The normal osmolality with a low $[Na^+]_p$ indicate normal concentration. The report of a "milky" plasma is the important clue, and it suggests a hyperlipoidemia. Determinations of plasma lipids should be made. See Chapter 3 for a discussion of this.

The other ions in plasma are decreased in concentration for the same reason. The simplest way of estimating what the concentration of the ions would be if the lipid did not take up such a large volume of the plasma is to assume that the $[Na^+]$ per volume of plasma water is within normal limits, since the osmolality is normal. The observed $[Na^+]$ is about 87% of normal. Corrections for $[HCO_3^-]$ and $[K^+]$ are:

For $[HCO_3^-]$ $\qquad 23 \times \dfrac{100}{87} \quad = \quad 26.5$ mEq/L

For $[K^+]$ $\qquad 3.3 \times \dfrac{100}{87} \quad = \quad 3.8$ mEq/L

The calculated values indicate what these values would be if the plasma were 92% water, instead of having its water content depressed by the lipids. These calculated values are in normal range.

Treatment

Since there is no disturbance of water balance, no treatment is necessary.

CASE 7

Diagnosis

1. Water deficit with hyperosmolality
2. Saltwater loss
3. Compensated respiratory acidosis, with a probable superimposed metabolic acidosis
4. Some K^+ deficit, but not sufficient to cause significant hypopotassemia
5. Normal magnesium concentration

Comment

1. The history of no food or water intake plus the plasma osmolality of 300 mOsm/kg water indicates a net loss of water.

The $[Na^+]_p$ and high urine specific gravity are consistent with this.

2. The history of diarrhea together with the findings of orthostatic hypotension, decreased skin turgor, and low body temperature all indicate a saltwater loss.

3. Chronic emphysema together with an elevated Pco_2, high $[HCO_3^-]_p$, and low pH establishes a respiratory acidosis with certainty. The $[HCO_3^-]$ is elevated more than would be predicted by the water deficit. The loss of high $[HCO_3^-]$ fluid in the stool would suggest an added metabolic acidosis. Starvation could add to this, but with no increase in the anion gap, this is not a factor.

4. Potassium salts are lost in the stools, but there has not been sufficient loss to move plasma K^+ out of normal limits. With the acidosis, K^+ has undoubtedly moved out of cells, but since it is unlikely that the respiratory acidosis will be reversed, K^+ will not move back into cells during treatment.

Treatment

1. Measures would be taken to control the diarrhea, but these are not considered here.

2. A hypotonic solution is necessary to replace the intracellular fluid volume deficit and increase milliosmolar concentration. This may be given as 5% glucose in water—with a probable volume of 3–4 liters—or as 4–6 liters of 1/2 strength lactated Ringer's solution so that ECF volume deficit is treated concomitantly. Isotonic lactated Ringer's solution may also be used following restitution of osmolar concentration to normal.

3. The amount of isotonic salt to be given intravenously is that volume needed to revert the clinical signs of ECF deficit to normal.

4. One should not attempt to return $[HCO_3^-]_p$ to normal values in this patient, because the elevation represents an important compensation for the respiratory acidosis.

5. No intensive therapy with either K^+ or Mg^{++} salts is indicated.

CASE 8

Diagnosis

1. Increased concentration
2. Saltwater deficit
3. Normal acid-base balance
4. Probable potassium deficit, but no hypopotassemia
5. Normal magnesium

Comment

1. The osmolality indicates that the plasma is hypertonic. The $[Na^+]_p$ is normal, but calculation of the contribution of the glucose to the osmolality is necessary for interpretation.

$$\frac{(1,490 - 100) \times 10}{180} = 78 \text{ mOsm/L due to increase in glucose}$$

$$\frac{78}{2} = 39 \text{ mEq of } Na^+ \text{ salts to be equivalent to glucose}$$

$$140 + 39 = 179 \text{ (equivalent value for } [Na^+]_p \text{ to reflect osmolality}$$

This calculation then confirms the existence of a milliosmolar concentration, or water deficit.
2. The decrease in ECF volume is evident from the blood pressure, the decrease in skin turgor, and the hypothermia. The saltwater loss occurs because sodium is lost in the urine as a result of the osmotic diuresis associated with the hyperglycemia.
3. The potassium is a high normal. Potassium is probably leaving the cells as glycogen is broken down, and then being excreted in the urine. When the glycogen is reformed in the cells, in response to insulin treatment, hypopotassemia is likely to result.

Treatment

1. The patient should receive insulin in adequate amounts.
2. The patient has a saltwater deficit, and needs an isotonic salt

solution. Lactated Ringer's solution is the choice, and initially it should be administered rapidly.

3. The patient has hypertonic body fluids. It must be recognized that insulin will lower the blood glucose and reduce the tonicity of the fluids, so that hypotonic fluids are not needed.

4. The patient will probably need more K^+ than in the Ringer's solution. When the K^+ level falls to low normal values, 20 mEq/L K^+ should be added to the IV fluids, and should be given at a rate of about 20 mEq/hour.

CASE 9

Diagnosis

1. Normal concentration
2. Normal ECF volume
3. Normal acid-base balance
4. Normal potassium
5. Hypomagnesemia

Comment

Magnesium has been lost by gastric suction and has not been replaced. The symptoms and signs related to the nervous system are classical for hypomagnesemia.

Treatment

1. Continue replacement of fluids lost by gastric suction.
2. Give, in addition, sufficient 5% glucose in water IV to replace insensible loss plus urine volume.
3. Magnesium sulfate must be administered, either intramuscularly, or with IV fluids. About 150 mEq would probably be needed, but therapy should be based on the observed $[Mg^{++}]$ of plasma determined during treatment.

CASE 10

Diagnosis

1. Normal concentration
2. Normal ECF volume
3. Compensated respiratory alkalosis
4. Normal potassium
5. Normal magnesium

Comment

The anemia has produced a tissue hypoxia which has driven respiration so that the Pco_2 has decreased. The respiratory alkalosis is compensated, as indicated by the reduction in $[HCO_3^-]_p$.

Treatment

1. The patient should receive iron therapy or transfusion to raise [Hb].
2. It is important not to attempt to raise the $[HCO_3^-]$ by treatment with either sodium lactate or sodium bicarbonate because this would make the alkalosis worse.
3. Find the site of bleeding, and apply specific therapy to stop this.

Index